When All Else Fails…

A journey into the heart with
Medical Intuition
And Metatronic Energy

By Carmel Bell
– Medical Intuitive and Metatronic Therapist

When all Else Fails…

Copyright © 2010 Carmel Bell
All rights reserved. No part of this publication may be reproduced, stored in a retrieval system or transmitted in any form or by any means, electronic, mechanical, photocopying, recording or otherwise, without the prior written permission of the publisher.

The information, views, opinions and visuals expressed in this publication are solely those of the author(s) and do not reflect those of the publisher. The publisher disclaims any liabilities or responsibilities whatsoever for any damages, libel or liabilities arising directly or indirectly from the contents of this publication.

A copy of this publication can be found in the National Library of Australia.

ISBN: 9781921681684

The information in this book is neither diagnostic nor treating any specific health challenges. It is sold with the understanding that the authors and publishers are not engaged in rendering medical, health or any other kind of personal, professional services in the book. The reader is responsible for seeing to and continuing any medical treatment and care as advised by their own medical, health or competent professionals. The author makes no claim, promises or guarantees. All material in this publication is for informational purposes only, and put forward to assist the individual in their personal development. Use of this material is the responsibility of the reader.

Published by Book Pal
www.bookpal.com.au

Medical Intuition and Metatronic Healing in practice and in life

For Bernie. With every breath I love you. I left because of others. I came back because of you.

For Harley, James, Jean-Luc and Roslin. I love you and I am proud of each of you. Travel well.

And Merrie. My friend.

Acknowledgements

With love and gratitude to Allan Standley, Enzo Tenuta, Sarah Allen, Katherine Yeowart, Michealle Jones, Alyce Chin, Jude Flood, Fiona Brown, Rob Yeowart and Jason Allen. True friends. Amicu certus in re incerta cernitur.

To my family, Mark J. Stokes, Jean Stokes, Mark A. Stokes, Margaret Stokes, Katherine Yeowart, Elizabeth Killingbeck and Sarah Allen. I would not change a single thing. Live long and prosper.

And also Jodam Allingam. Family comes to us.

To Christine Taranto, Vicki Kapo, Louise Soltau, Piera Perri and Melanie Mitsios for guarding the fort and continuing to light the way.

To Gary Easte, Steve Tanner and Scott Hardy. Thank you for every compression, and for your compassion.

To Barb Stone, Jenny Altermatt and Libby Dartez. Without your enduring support and belief this journey may have been made, but it would have been lonely.

To Dr Rita Louise MI – for friendship given and received.

To Paula Hardgrave. For phonecalls and love.

To Devi and Debbie and the team at Bookpal for making this such a pleasant, easy experience.

To PMH Atwater who answered every question.

To Nanci Danison for her insight and friendship.

And to Melissa Hocking, for the hand of friendship and the disclaimer both. A true highlander.

For Peter, Hiram and Alexander who have all danced, laughed and cried with me.

For Metatron – for his endurance, tolerance, compassion and interference.

I would like to acknowledge all those people who have trusted in me and my abilities. Without your support there would have been no journey.

And also thank you to all those Medical Doctors, Pharmacists and Scientists and other health care professionals who trusted in what I have been given enough to help their clients.

We are a team, the finest team.

And finally, to those people who allowed me to share their journey with the readers of this book. Even in disguise, with dark glasses and false moustaches on, you are each of you a fascination into the depths of the human soul. Watching each of you grow and heal has helped heal me. Thank you.

"Circumstances do not make the man, they reveal him."
- James Allen

Contents

Medical Intuition and Metatronic Healing in practice and in life iii

Acknowledgements v

Chapter One: Introduction 1

Chapter Two: Deciding not to die 9

Chapter Three: Being the Medical Intuitive 33

Chapter Four: The who and the why. A job description 47

Chapter Five: The blocks to healing 72

Chapter Six: Finding out why 80

Chapter Seven: The art of Healing (the what) 86

Chapter Eight: Seeing Energy 96

Chapter Nine: Feeling Energy 113

Chapter Ten: Grounding and Sealing 117

Chapter Eleven: Metatronic Energy - an experiment . 122

Chapter Twelve: The Patterns 132

Chapter Thirteen: Self Healing 192

Chapter fourteen: Meetings with Metatron 205

Chapter fifteen: Removing stories 228

Chapter Sixteen: Waking up dead 251

Chapter Seventeen: Heaven 261

Chapter Eighteen: Re-entry 305

Chapter Nineteen: The side effects of Dying 318

Chapter Twenty: The Journey home 342

Index of Exercises 354

Bibliography 355

Chapter One:

Introduction

"What lies behind us and before us are tiny matters compared to what lies within us." - **Ralph Waldo Emerson**

My name is Carmel Bell and I am a Medical Intuitive. I have practiced Medical Intuition professionally since 1985 and in that time I have seen more than 10,000 clients. Today I am one of the most recognized founders of Medical Intuition. I am considered to be one of the top 10 Medical Intuitives in the world, which is a real honor. To know that so many people have trusted my skills and relied on my ability, from laymen to medical practitioners, is a privilege beyond description.

In this book you will find some of the cases that I have worked on, but you will also find the tale of my most difficult client ever – me.

People contact me for many reasons; reasons that are physical, emotional *and* spiritual. There is no set reason that people *seem* to contact me, there is no set client type and every story is unique. I have often thought about my clients, wondering if there was one thing in common that brings them to my door.

The answer is yes, there is a common theme. It is a question and it is the same question that I asked myself – 'What is wrong with me?'

I have seen people from just about every profession, from housewives to prostitutes, priests to professional criminals. And yet they all come with this one question in common – they are asking what is wrong with them, why they are not well.

And there is also one common answer, one common theme.

None of them are settled or peaceful inside their heart – inside their emotional heart. Within their heart they hold secrets and discontentedness, anger, sorrow or secret longings. They hold resentments and hurts and because of what their heart is containing, they become ill. Inside of them they hold a heart of darkness that will not let them be easy. And their body is displaying what their heart is feeling. Bent over *is* overburdened.

Simply put, very few people are *true* to themselves. Their battle between their heart and what is *expected* of them, by themselves and by others, becomes overwhelming. They come to see me when *all else* has failed.

Each of us could be forgiven for thinking that it is surely the easiest task in the world - to be true to you, to know what you want, to know what you should do and then to do it. But it is the most difficult task of all. Do you really know what you want? Really? What about when you are told that you need to choose between your family of birth or your husband? Your house or the new one interstate? Your body will reflect every conundrum that you experience; no matter how well you hide it.

A Medical Intuitive is the person you call when you are feeling lost, when you ask yourself – what is wrong with me? What is hidden in my heart and in my body that I cannot see?

Medical Intuitives are the cartographers who read the map of your body and of your energy system.

To try and explain to you fully what Medical Intuition is at best a time consuming task and at worst, a lecture. It is better to lead you on a journey into my world and to show you some of the extraordinary and *ordinary* cases I have been involved with.

I diagnose the energy system using intuition and knowledge and I call this skill set Medical Intuition and I also heal people using an incredible energy frequency that has been gifted to me by the Archangel Metatron. My story and Metatron are inexorably entwined.

I will walk you through some of my life in this book to show you how I discovered Metatronic Energy and how I simultaneously discovered Medical Intuition alongside this energy.

Not all Medical Intuitives are healers and not all people who use Metatronic Energy are Medical Intuitives. I am quite unique in that I am both. This is how I work and this is what I teach.

I truly love this profession. I feel at my best when I work as a Medical Intuitive. I have seen many fabulous results, both from the diagnosis – as it helps people to know what is the matter with them and what they may need to do to rectify that and also from the healings. Metatronic Energy has saved the life, the sanity and the hope of thousands of people. It has saved my life, so I can speak confidently from personal experience. I would *not* be alive and working today if it were not for my own profession.

Medical Intuition is not the kind of skill that should be taught through a book alone, any more than surgery should. It is something that should be passed on, hand to hand, demonstrated and nurtured because it requires practice, commitment and endurance, so I will tell you about what I do and how I do it and I will teach you about energy, how to see it and how to feel it. But the true in-depth learning, I will save for when we meet face to face.

What you will learn is how a Medical Intuitive works, so that you know what to expect if you need to see one, how to see and manage energy for yourself, both Bio-energy and Metatronic Energy and how to heal yourself. You are the only healer who can heal yourself, despite what people may say. Healing requires complicity and co-operation. Both are in your hands.

This is the story of my life. This is the story of how I became a Medical Intuitive and it is the story of what I do every day, week after week, year after year.

A brief personal biography

I first died when I was four-years-old. In that brief NDE I met Jesus and an Archangel called Metatron. I had no idea who Metatron was, or was meant to be. I just talked to him because he was there, with Jesus. I knew who Jesus was because my parents were Catholic.

At that time I wanted to be a doctor but Metatron told me I would not be. He told me that instead I would do this – Medical Intuition – and use his energy to do it. Metatron 'gave' this energy to me and I returned to life with his energy on my hand.

Being four I did very little with his energy until I died again during an operation when I was 17. During that NDE I re-met Metatron and Jesus. They told me that I had made a few wrong turns in my life so far and they redirected me back towards Medical Intuition.

I spent the next few years learning and practicing what I thought was the right thing to do, in between running a successful dress-making business for myself.

Over the years I found that challenges kept being thrown at me that kept placing me back on this path. At one time it was suggested by a doctor that I may have lung cancer because I was so unwell and I was smoking. I listened to him, thanked him and left his office, never returning. Instead I sorted out my life and used Metatronic Energy to heal myself.

But I did not realize until about 1985 when I was learning clairvoyance, that what I was doing – combining my intuitive skills with the medical knowledge that I had taught myself – was my calling. I was actually doing what I had been told I would by Metatron, but without realizing it. The moment I made that realization, I started working in this profession consciously. I was excited, but I was also afraid. I had never even heard of Edgar Cayce. Caroline Myss was still unknown of. I was on my own. But I was driven.

I found myself being a Medical Intuitive on the side, keeping it quiet and yet becoming busier and busier until Medical Intuition took over. I coined the phrase Aura Diagnostician to describe my profession and in 1993 opened up my own clinic.

By 1994 I was busier than ever and then in 1996 Caroline Myss published her signature book – '*Anatomy of Spirit'* – and the groundswell started to grow rapidly. It was then that people started to call me a Medical Intuitive.

I have always been busy and by 1994 I had a number of medical practitioners who were clients and who referred clients to me, but there was something more that I wanted. I wanted Medical Intuition, as it was called since Myss's book, to be medically and socially accepted. I was just not sure about what I could use to progress Medical Intuition. I had never seen a miraculous, instantaneous healing and as every piece of literature remotely connected to something like this seemed to include that, I was feeling pretty flat.

In 1999 I diagnosed myself with a brain tumor and Cushing's disease and had it confirmed medically. Despite now having this awful disease, I kept very well, fit and thin for a person with Cushing's.

Then in 2007 I realized I was going to die but I knew it was not from the brain tumor. I was told by my guides that my heart was going to fail even though I could not find anything wrong with my heart. I was puzzled. I told my doctor and she organized a halter monitor to be put on me so that they could test my heart, but everything seemed normal on the test. Even so, the warnings continued to increase.

Despite the brain tumor and Cushing's disease, I was still very fit, running each day for about half an hour and working for hours every day with clients.

Although I had been teaching weekend workshops in Metatronic Energy and Medical Intuition since 1995, I had not yet taught anyone to be a Medical Intuitive. But knowing I was going to die I decided that I should teach some people to practice the way I do. I wanted to pass this on.

I started my college in 2008 and within a month of announcing it I was full with enrolments. I chose the 20 best students and I began to teach, developing the course as I went, with Bernie, my husband, who is an ambulance paramedic and university lecturer. We also had other medical practitioners come in to teach.

The first course finished in December 2008 and I finally agreed to have the brain tumor removed. I was now very tired and it was finally starting to show.

The brain surgery was successful but I awoke from surgery still knowing I was going to die. I told Bernie and again I told my doctor but there seemed to be nothing any of us could do. There was nothing wrong with me.

On February 15th 2009, I died.

During my sleep I had a sudden cardiac arrest for unknown causes. Bernie found me and he saved me but it took him and six other paramedics 47 minutes to bring me back. I was severely brain damaged with global brain damage caused by Hypoxic Brain Injury.

Fortunately I had access to Metatronic Energy because I used it on myself, by myself, to restore my brain back to normal. That is all that was used on my brain. There is no therapy for brain damage.

When I recovered reasonably from brain damage I realized that I did have the extraordinary case I felt I had been missing; I had me.

Now, I thought, maybe it was time to write about Medical Intuition and Metatronic Energy, to talk to you about what it can do and what it feels like. Metatronic

Energy is a remarkable, clean, simple and powerful energy. It saved me. Medical Intuition is brilliant at finding the way through all the trouble. Between the two of them, they work well.

Chapter Two:

Deciding not to die

"The greatest mistake in the treatment of diseases is that there are physicians for the body and physicians for the soul, although the two cannot be separated." - **Plato**

Carla – throat cancer

> *Dear Carmel,*
> *I have throat cancer. A friend of mine told me about you and I am contacting you because I am desperate. Next week I have to go to hospital to have radiation therapy and I am scared. My oncologist has told me that if we cannot put this into remission that I only have a short time left to live. I want to live.*
> *I am hoping you can help me.*
> *Thank you,*
> *Carla*

I saw Carla shortly after I received that email, within a month. She had already started radiation therapy and when she came in she was barely able to talk. She sounded breathless and she had to hold her throat each time she spoke. She carried water and a straw with her everywhere as she could only sip a little through the straw. Carla was painfully thin and clearly in distress.

She wanted to know if the treatment was working, what she had done to create throat cancer and was the cancer in retreat or going somewhere else in her body.

I could see from her energy that she was nearly at the end of her journey. Carla was running on pure will power. The radiation treatment was not yet working and unless something shifted in her, it probably never would. There just was not enough reason for her to live.

Beneath the gauntness of her skin you could see she was a beautiful woman, but she looked like she had been eaten alive, from the inside out.

The medical prognosis for her was also not good. Her oncologist was going to give this next therapy a shot and if that did not work then there was not much else he felt they could do.

We sat and talked, which was a little difficult given how hard it was for her to speak. Carla would gasp for air, speak softly until the air ran out and then gasp again. It was painful to watch, but nonetheless, we did okay. I asked her about her life, how she felt about it, how she got on with her family, her husband and her children. Then I asked her what she wanted to do with her life.

Carla did not feel that she had ever done what she wanted to do. She had married young and put her life on hold to help her husband develop their business, then they had had two children together and again Carla had sacrificed her wants for the needs of her children. When her children were older, her parents had needed her help whilst her father was dying, but he had died two years before and now her mother was elderly and living alone. Within weeks of her father dying, Carla had been diagnosed with cancer. She was also her mother's main support, although she herself was so sick. In short, in all of Carla's 53 years, she felt that she had not yet lived her own life.

Carla was married to Rob, whom she loved but felt strongly disempowered by. He earned the money and had built her a beautiful home, but it was the home *he* wanted, where *he* wanted it and not where or how Carla had wanted it. Although Carla liked her house, it was not what she would have chosen. Carla was *secretly* quite angry with Rob. She felt that Rob did not seem to like anything she did and judged her wants to be a waste of time - even if he never said it, he certainly acted like it, she said. He liked her to be there and available for him.

Carla had been close to her father, but she was not emotionally close to her mother, feeling more like a servant, so she felt lost to her family.

Her children were living out of home and they hardly came home to visit and Carla had been feeling lost and unvalued by them as well for quite some time. She expressed that she no longer knew what she wanted to do, but she knew she did not want to do what she was doing. She wanted more fun. It seemed to her that she was dying and no-one was even noticing.

Upon further discussion it became quite clear that Carla felt as if her husband had taken her away from all her family and her friends – they lived quite a distance out of town – and this meant she was isolated and relying on him, but he did not want to spend much time with her, he was caught up at work all the time. He was probably scared, watching the woman he loved being consumed by a disease he could not beat. Regardless, Carla felt trapped and disempowered and now she was wondering what the point of life was. Throat cancer was her way out. No-one could blame her if she died, but Carla had just lately realized that she wanted to live.

The throat chakra is our communication centre. It is where we express all that we feel, whether that feeling is anger, love, success or anything else. Carla had spent all her life not being able to say what it was she wanted. She reasoned that her time would come, but it had not. She was free, freer than she had ever been with the children out of home, her father dead and she was financially well off. But in effect, Carla was still a servant and a child. Worse, she felt she was voiceless and without the right to 'vote' about her own life.

Although Carla had not yet realized this was what was killing her, she did very quickly see it after we talked about her issues. I shared my insights into what had caused the cancer; we talked about what could be done about it. I explained that we would need to rattle issues through her system but she would still need the radiation therapy. We needed to move the creating energies out of her so that she was free to choose where she would go from here. I felt confident that between her oncologist and me, we could make a real win for Carla.

Carla was despairing but she trusted what I was telling her. She was only expected to live a few more weeks, so there was not a lot to lose. I felt sure that I could get her a lot more life than a few weeks and a life with quality.

Carla sat on the small stool that I used for my healings and I dropped the energy that I use – Metatronic Energy – through her. A few minutes later I was finished. The Metatronic Energy would run now without me and it would continue on for at least three weeks, without any intervention – longer it Carla could manage her energy properly.

I explained to Carla how she needed to manage the results and then we rescheduled a follow-up appointment for after her radiation therapy session. To me, energetically Carla was looking much better. I could see shifts occurring in her already and I was feeling hopeful.

(email received one month after treatment)

Dear Carmel,
I cannot believe the difference that I am feeling. I am sleeping really well and I am happy. I have moved part-time into the unit that we own in Warrandyte so now I can easily see my friends and my family. Rob stays with me on the weekends and we go out together. I feel like I have a life. I am still having the radiation therapy and my oncologist is hopeful that this is now actually working. Thank you so much. I will see you in a few weeks.
Love Carla

Carla came back to see me about a month after the email. She was thinner than ever and she reported that her throat was burnt and frequently bled, but when I looked at her, energetically it appeared the cancer was on the retreat. I told her what I was seeing and that I felt hopeful for her future. We again talked about what she wanted from her life and she mentioned that she would like to be well enough to go overseas.

She was still in the unit, and Rob was there full-time for the moment, looking after her. Despite all the pain in her throat, she was feeling fantastic – even if eating was harder than ever. She did tell me that the oncologist was pleased with the results so far – it was better than expected.

I treated her again with the Metatronic Energy and I asked Carla to keep me informed about her progress as I felt she did not need any more treatments from me for now.

(email received about one year after treatment)

Dear Carmel,
I thought I would let you know that all signs of the cancer seem to be gone for now. I still have trouble swallowing and I have to have regular check-ups. But I feel a lot more hopeful. My oncologist thinks that we may have beaten this and he is amazed. Rob and I are very happy and we are planning a holiday together. Thank you so much for your help.
Love Carla.

Carla is now recovering from throat cancer. She still has problems with swallowing and drinking but she assures me that she improves all the time, becoming happier and healthier.

We had one more session after that last email so that I could assess the likely future progress and from what I could see, Carla no longer had cancer cells in her body.

There was no 'one moment' that happened in my life to make me a Medical Intuitive. For me, absolutely every moment, including now, is about learning to be a Medical Intuitive and it has been about practicing and living by the qualities and the moral code of a Medical Intuitive. It is cases like Carla's that keep me going and keep me learning.

Every moment of my life, from my birth, to who my parents were, to my siblings, to the places I have lived has been about this path. It is impossible to separate the moments, relegating this moment to that section and that other moment to something else. With a profession such as a Medical Intuitive, you either are one, or you are not – 100%.

A lot of people do not really know what Medical Intuition is, or what it may be used for. Most people who pick up a book like this do so for one of a few reasons.

1: Because they are ill, or someone they love is ill and all else has failed to give them what they need.

2: It is something they would like to experience for themselves.

3: It is something they would like to learn.

4: It is something they feel they may already be doing, but want to check. They want to see how I do what I do and what the difference is for them.

This book is for all those people. I hope to show you and educate you about Medical Intuition. To try and actually teach you Medical Intuition in a book would be irresponsible of me. It is a serious profession, with real responsibilities and consequences. It requires hands on teaching.

The Basic components required for Medical Intuition

Below are some good, common sense pieces of advice that you may need, whether you are seriously looking at training as a Medical Intuitive or just want to know more about how we work so that you can decide if it something that might help you.

Use this information as a way to assess any Medical Intuitive that you see. This, and a referral from a trusted source, is your best protection.

Because Medical Intuition and alternative healing in general is often so untrained and largely unregulated, you need to maintain commonsense practices when dealing with a therapist. For instance, an energy practitioner will not need to have you undress, but a massage or physical therapist may require you to. Maintain your sense of self and your boundaries. Believe what is believable and remember that the human body does not heal instantaneously. Even if the energy to make it heal is there, the cells themselves take time to alter. You will not walk out 'cured' from anywhere.

I hope this book will give you some idea as to what is involved with Medical Intuition. It is a fantastic, exciting and exhilarating profession and it does require teaching.

How can Medical Intuition help you?

The human body is a finely tuned machine, balanced between all of its components. The human brain can process more information than any computer yet invented and the human body can achieve feats that are still impossible with current robotics technology. If something gets thrown out of balance in you, everything else is placed at risk. For example, deplete your potassium stores and you can suffer a sudden cardiac arrest. If you drop your iron levels too low, you will be fighting for breath and for energy. Make yourself sad and you will struggle to even stand upright. Lift a weight that is too heavy and damage your spine and you may not even be able to walk. The body has a resilience that is unbeatable, but it is fragile.

Emotions can destroy as easily as drugs. Bully a child and the results can be long-term and terrible. People do die of a broken heart. So much of what can, and does, go wrong with the body is untestable and untreatable by conventional means until it becomes really gross. In other words, very few professions can even see, let alone remove the second head on your shoulder until the second grows there.

Medical Intuition can often see the 'second head'. By using Medical Intuition you can see inside your body and look for problems that are there but too fine or small to be seen by conventional means. A well trained Medical Intuitive can see if you are low in a vitamin or mineral – and why you are low.

Everybody who is unwell *knows* when they are unwell. It is a very rare person who genuinely does not have any idea of when they are sick. Most of us know but we don't know what to do about it.

Medical Intuition is designed to discover the undiscoverable, to go into the world of the unknown and to chart it.

I know that many people will think to themselves: "This is bound to be complicated and difficult, or I need to be special to use it." No it isn't. The basic components that you need to work on yourself are fairly easy.

If you want to treat other people it is more complicated because you need to be able to understand them. But you *already* understand you. You just need to learn what to do with your energy system to keep it safe and operating at an optimal level.

The Soul and Spiritual Guidance

As an Intuitive I am dealing with the soul, mine and yours and I am working with Guides.

If *you* want to work with Guides, I would recommend that you find a teacher to help you to communicate with your Guides as you will only be as good as you and your Guides become together. So find the best teacher you can and learn to listen to your Guides. I promise you; very few guides will call you 'beloved' or say things like 'We of the Atlantian people's council...' Guides are real and sensible. They will talk to you about the things that matter to you, now, today. And in my experience most of them also have a sense of humour.

If you are hearing guidance and your guides are sounding overly grandiose, please be cautious.

I have known quite a few Medical Intuitives who have not used overtly or knowingly, Spiritual Guides to help them. You may find that you never do, either. But I would encourage you to look a little further and see if that quiet knowing is not coming from a Spirit Guide. After all, they are in Heaven and Heaven is right here. You are in Heaven now, just in a different dimension.

The Body

A Medical Intuitive is looking after the body so naturally it is wisdom for a Medical Intuitive to have a good understanding of anatomy and physiology. If you see a Medical Intuitive and they are asking you where the liver is, you should probably have a little concern.

Don't be afraid to do a bit of research about the Medical Intuitive you wish to see.

I have been learning about the complexities of the inter-relationship of mind, body and spirit and the effect of emotion on the body all my life.

I have learned that everything *is* energy and I have learned how to influence energy to facilitate healing at the deepest and most profound level. To do this I have had to learn about the body and the ailments that afflict it, in heart and mind and body, as well as about the medicines and herbs that you can take, if you need them. All of these learnings are ongoing and I have had fantastic and patient teachers, assisting me in my path.

Just like a piece of coal forms into a diamond by being hidden in the dark and compressed by unbelievable pressure, so too does a Medical Intuitive go through trial by 'fire', again and again. I have never met a 'born' Medical Intuitive who has not had to make that journey. I think this is because the forces in heaven charged us with a mission – to bring to Humanity the skills needed to energetically heal the body and to lead the way so that others – you - can learn.

Science

Science has given us the tools and the knowledge to understand a great deal of the working of the body, but even with the outstanding knowledge we have access to, we have been – until now – unable to recognize that there is another aspect to the human body which has an enormous effect on the body's ability to function, or not. This is why research continues all the time into how the body works, why it works and what causes it to fail.

Frequently though, the spirit is still overlooked, but without that 'spark' nothing else works.

What drives us to achieve? What makes us curl up and die when distressed? People genuinely do die of a broken heart. Our spirit defines us, yet we are unable to measure that definition by any *machine* we currently have.

Medicine

Most Medical Intuitives have a good and close affiliation with doctors, for good reason. We work really well together, hand in hand. I love Western Medicine. I think it is fantastic and it has saved many lives. A lot of people in alternative professions speak disparagingly of Western Medicine and science, which is a pity because 'Western' Medicine was alternative once, also. We need both.

It is usually quite okay and even helpful to use alternative and western together. Don't be afraid to discuss this with your doctor, if you need to.

Medical Intuitives

There is nothing that can go wrong within the body that is a mystery unable to be unravelled. It just takes a little bit of hunting and looking and that is what Medical Intuition does.

We are the machines that can see the 'will to live'. We are the machines that see the broken heart and also see the reason for the broken heart and then set about fixing it.

The Human body is the living, breathing embodiment of your existence, your thoughts, your feelings, your past, your future, the food you have eaten and even the food your ancestors have eaten.

I once heard it said about a scientist that he was 'quite a man' because he still went to church. He believed in a force greater than science. Science and spirit are a lot more closely aligned than we have allowed.

Scientists like to test, prove, or disprove everything and that is fantastic. We are as advanced as we are because of science. I know that in the future scientists will be able to test many things that are considered spiritual and therefore are currently untestable. Scientists will eventually test them, prove them and include them into their laws.

Spirit also tests everything. The existence of something; some thought, some concept and some idea will eventually prove its existence because the 'thing' will be created. Every invention started as nothing more than a thought. As Descartes said – 'I think, therefore I am.' If you can think about something, it can become real. Asimov and his laws of robotics are a case in point. Issac Asimov wrote a book called '*I, Robot*", written in the 50's where robots were basically fantasy and now humanoid robots are a reality and they are applying Asimov's robot laws to the development of robots. His thoughts and ideas eventually became a reality.

Now apply this point to the fear of developing cancer...

I know that it is difficult for some scientists to reconcile the spiritual. I also know that it is incredulous for to those who practice spirituality to accept that scientists could fail to see what was right in front of their eyes. Science can tell us that the heart beats. But why did the heart start to beat? And sometimes why does it continue to beat long after it should have stopped? Or resume beating long after it did stop? Or continue to beat even after life has become too intolerable for a body to breathe? What is it that makes the heart continue?

Spirit.

Spirit is the great unknown. It is the answer to the question of the meaning of life.

This is a book about spirit. And spirit is not as far away from you as you might believe. In fact, it is right here, next to you, right now.

You don't need a priest to tell you how to live. You just have to be a compassionate human. You really just have to say to yourself 'Would I be happy if someone broke into my house and stole my things?' or 'Would I be happy if someone beat my sister, killed my cat, stole my wallet, ran into my car and then drove away?' Perhaps you might be saying, 'Maybe I would love it if someone was rude to me when I was trying to do my job.'

The lesson is to treat other people how you would like to be treated, only better, sooner and more often. Not hard is it?

Being the healer

You may think that a healer has no problems. Or you may believe that the more a healer suffers, the better they must be. Both beliefs are true and both are false. The human experience means that our body will become the record for our biography. Your story is written in every cell of your being. Every moment matters because everything you hear, think, feel, eat, read, see and do will be recorded somewhere in your body. It is also known and acknowledged that a lot of what your relatives eat and do will also have been stored in your body. This is a field called Epigenetics. Every moment matters. You cannot hide from your family – they go with you wherever you go.

Your biography will become your biology. You are a walking book. I am a book reader.

Healing yourself

No human, no healer needs to cling to their illness to be good at their job. Learn that. Do not cling to your pain. Let it go. Forgive yourself. One of my favourite sayings is "There but for the grace of God, go I." Once, when I was at one of the lowest moments of my life, a man that I barely knew said that to me. The person quoting that to me allowed me to breathe again and to recover from a situation I never thought I could.

There, but for the grace of God, go I.

The realisation that we all, not just the young, make mistakes. To have the compassion to see beyond the mistakes others make is a gift and a blessing. I know that I would not want to be viewed in the same light as I was when I was 15, 20 or even 30. Come to think of it, 40 was a pretty terrible time, too! To have the compassion to see beyond the mistakes that we ourselves make, is a necessity. More often than not, people lack compassion for themselves.

Compassion

One of the greatest gifts that you can give to someone else is the gift of compassion. Most of my life has also been spent learning compassion. To learn about the body was a necessary task, but it was the easier task because the body stays fairly fixed – two arms, two legs, a head and the internal organs.

But compassion depends on *you*, your experiences, your ability to feel and to not judge. Compassion will depend on your ability to let people tell you anything and have you *not* reel around in horror or tell them that they are wrong to feel that way. That is a real gift – to them and to you.

So although Medical Intuition is an intuitive skill that does not mean that it is an untrained or untested skill.

A Medical Intuitive has a responsibility, just as everybody does who wishes to title themselves a healer and that is to be as healthy and as self aware as possible.

You really should not be traipsing about in someone else's heart without first examining your own.

And that does not mean that you cannot do this if you are not 100% well. You can, but you need to be aware that you are not well and why you are not well. You need to be prepared to examine your life from every angle, every day, but without becoming boring about it. Not everybody will want to do this and they don't have to.

Medical Intuition is a fantastic profession – a real cross between complementary and traditional medicine, if done properly. It helps more people than any other profession I have ever personally witnessed and it does no harm whilst doing it. It uses no drugs, no medicines and requires absolutely nothing secret.

There is never a moment when I am *not* a Medical Intuitive, no matter what I am doing. You talk to me; you are talking to an MI. It never turns off. Just remember that this is not all I am, it is just some of what I am.

Integrity

Whenever you offer healing to another person, or even just lend them an ear, it is crucial that you keep a sense of integrity with you. Integrity is a deep sense of honesty and truthfulness in regard to the motivation of your actions. It is doing the right thing because the right thing is the right thing to do. Make no promises you cannot keep.

Discretion and other good manners

Always maintain confidentiality.

Never divulge without permission.

Always keep in close touch with a client's primary care physician.

Never dispense advice that you are not sure of.

Curing

You cannot cure everyone. Not everyone can be healed and that is okay. Dying is a part of life. Ill health is inevitable. Some of the loveliest people I have met have had the worst health and some of the most bitter or angry people have been hale and hearty, right up to the moment they died.

Using energy – performing a healing

Energy moves in an instant. The longer you take to run energy into a person, even yourself, does not make the energy better or more effective. When I 'heal' someone, I will only run energy for a few short minutes.

People are also never disrobed in a session with me; they are never lying down, but sit on a stool, always. There is no haunting melody playing and no pungent incense. So many people have allergies that my space is as scent free as possible. I touch people only twice – on the shoulders to let them know I am beginning and to let them know I am finishing the session. I don't sing, chant or dance about.

Always test energy and your methods. Make sure that what you are doing is necessary and not just superstition. Energy works because energy works. It runs in a certain way – from right to left actually. That is science.

Be gentle with you. We are all of us in the gutter, but some of us are looking at the stars. (*Oscar Wilde*)

Client: female 44 – left breast cancer and bladder cancer

October '08- Katie came to see me because she was dying and she knew it. Her oncologist had told her that she had only a few options left but that they could still perform a radical procedure.

She came to see me because she had decided that she wanted to live. But what was there for Katie to live for? She had no children of her own, she disliked her job and wanted to break up with her partner. Her partner was impotent and they never slept together anyway.

Her oncologist had everything under control physically. There were no parasites that I could see in Katie's body, her magnesium levels were okay – in short, despite the cancer she looked okay, but it was easy to see that she was dying. There was a deep sadness and dissatisfaction in Katie and it showed in the way she sat slightly hunched, in the way she dressed all in white and grey and the way that she spoke in a fairly flat monotone. I could get her to laugh occasionally, though. Her cancer, for a woman with such a healthy lifestyle, was particularly aggressive.

What I could see was that Katie had a secret. I watched her energy system for a while as we talked, expecting something huge, but it was nothing.

Katie smoked.

Her family would be mortified if they knew. Her partner was not around her enough to know she smoked and you and I might think that this was such a non event secret that why would anyone mind? But Katie was meant to be the good girl and she smoked. It was representative of many things in her life that were wrong, all the different areas that she hid herself from people, that she lied about. There was no-one that Katie was honest with, no-one that she told the truth to, or really loved. She was not close to her sisters either and she had a cat which she did not like.

Katie was dying and she would be dead within three months, I thought, if she did not change her life around.

She was shocked when I confronted her with her secret, but also relieved as now we could talk about it. I knew that her smoking meant she was angry with her father, I knew that the cancer was because of the dysfunction in her relationship with her mother and I knew that if I could get Katie to acknowledge this, we had a chance of her recovering.

I talked to Katie about the patterns I was seeing and how they affected her. We ran the energy through her body and I taught her how to manage the results. I was reasonably confident that many issues would shift and shift quickly. I told her that there was nothing and no-one at fault for her disease, that there was nothing to get over, but that she needed to assume responsibility for her illness before she could get well. In other words, stop blaming the world, and get on with it instead. At first Katie argued with me, then she understood what I was saying and it all made sense. She was not at fault, she was not to blame but she was in charge.

I disconnected her from her parents and from her boyfriend but I left the cat alone. We all need something to love and then I asked her to contact me in a month with a report.

A month later Katie contacted me to let me know she was still alive and feeling better. She was getting on better with her parents and was even planning on spending Christmas with them. She and the cat were also feeling happier. She had told her parents that she smoked but they had been okay with it and she had also broken up with her boyfriend.

Katie was feeling hopeful. We used Metatronic Energy on her again, working on losing the belief that she was better off being miserable and then she went off to live.

December 2009 – Katie contacted me for another session. She was still not smoking, still single and had finished all her treatment. There was no sign of the cancer that I could see. Katie was happy.

Even when you are dying, you will struggle for life and if the right key is found, you will live. Katie needed some integrity in her life. She needed honesty and love. She needed to lose the anger she was carrying and the guilt. We are all of us humans, all of us are in the gutter, but some of us are looking at the stars.

Exercise:

Decide how you want to live your life. Make a conscious choice. It can be simple, and in fact it should be simple. Also aim for something *not* altruistic. We are not looking for the next Gandhi, we are looking for the next you – the real you. Of course, you may have already found you, and if you have, congratulations!

But for the rest of us ... what do you want your life to be like? What do you want from life? You *pay attention* to what really matters, not to what you say matters. For instance, if you say, "Yeah, I love riding motor bikes!" but you have not ridden for 20 years because your partner does not want you to or you can't afford it or *any* other reason, I am going to tell you, you don't really care about it. You only *want* to care about it.

So – our list ... what do you want in your life?
> More fun?
> More time to read?
> More success?
> Less guilt?
> To be healthy in my body and my mind?
> To find love?
> To find peace?
> More friends?

Your task is to find out what you want. Look for what is simple and look to what the patterns are in your life. What are these patterns telling you?

When All Else Fails

Find out what really matters to you and decide if this is what you want to matter to you.

If it does not matter, you will not give it any time, even if you want it to matter.

Chapter Three:

Being the Medical Intuitive

"A healing occurs when one knows one's connection to the entire fabric of the Universe" - **Bertrand Russell**

Health is a decision.

You are the products of your thought and your beliefs. Change your thoughts and you can change the world. You will *definitely* change you. If you are unwell or unhappy it is because you believe something. That 'something' may be a belief that you are stuck or helpless or that everyone hates you or that you are worthless. No matter what your thoughts are, they will affect your health.

You can change your thoughts.

A lot of people have their own ideas on what makes a good MI, or a good session. I'm often confused. I think you might be, too.

Some Medical Intuitives are full of dietary advice, whilst others espouse exercise as the key and a few tout religions as the way to enlightenment.

Religion is not part of this. Spirit is.

Drugs are not part of this. Science is.

"None so virtuous as a reformed whore." It is an old saying and it is very definitely a truism. Anyone who converts to a way of life is bound to be more fanatical than someone who has lived that way *all* their life. The way that I practice Medical Intuition has been my way, all my life.

My advice to you is to trust yourself.

Most people who end up here reading a book on a skill like Medical Intuition do so because they or someone they love are ill or unhappy. Other people end up here because they have a desire to help people. Whatever your reason, I intend to try to help you understand what it is like *to be* a Medical Intuitive and whether or not this field is something you may like to explore.

I understand what it is like to be seriously ill or very unhappy. I know how desperate you can become for answers when you or someone you love is ill or dying and no-one can give you what you need – help.

I understand what it is like to stand in a dark place. I know, because I have been there, in the dark, walking in circles, crying and praying to God for help and feeling unanswered. I know what it is like to have a heart so heavy that I feel I cannot live another minute, another second.

I have been in the dark wood, wandering alone and I know the path. I can lend you the map, if you wish.

It is in a drawer marked 'You need to have fun and follow your heart.'

In Botswana they have a saying, "To look into the heart of another is to look into the wilderness."

Every moment matters. I would like to share with you something that I discovered. It is that you will find truth and spirituality in every moment, under every rock, behind every bush, in every song playing, every book being read. Truth and spirituality is everywhere.

I used to think you needed to read books like the Bible to find wisdom and then I noticed that wisdom was everywhere and that what I needed to find or hear would be wherever my attention was. Truth is everywhere. Spirit is everywhere.

You are already a fully developed spirit. You are here, on earth, to learn to be *human*.

There is not one moment that is more important than any other moment in your life, nor is there any book that holds more messages for you, when you are looking for help, than any other. If you are drawn to it, it will have something in there for you.

I can lend you the map but I cannot let you off the hook. There will still be grief and sorrow and anger and joy. Yes, you will still dance and sing and yell. You will still cry, laugh, live and die, because you are human.

If you never felt loss, how would you know joy when you found something or someone?

If you never felt pain at your mistreatment, would you recognize kindness?

What about rejection and acceptance? Or wealth and poverty? Everything needs to be felt and experienced so that you will know how to enjoy your life.

And here is another secret. The difference between feeling pain and having fun is often as simple as choice. If you are driving a car downhill when the brakes suddenly fail, you have two choices. You can panic, scream a lot and pray, or you can kick back, relax and enjoy the ride. Yes, I know – crazy thought, but you would probably be dead anyway, so why not have fun before you die. Take with you the memory of laughter.

Below are some of the lessons and advice that I pass on to my clients in session with them. I like to teach people to have fun. I even call my workshops 'Fun-shops'.

I never saw the sense to work when I could have fun. You can perform your job with a lot of joy, have fun and still get the job done, if you want to.

There is no problem, no task, which is so onerous that you have to add misery. Or so I think. Read this ...

... *"The solution to every problem is simple. It is the space in between wherein the mystery lies."*

The solution to every problem is simple.

It is the SPACE in between wherein the mystery lies.

Beautiful isn't it? It is simple and direct.

Let's say that the problem is that you have a disease and the solution is you need for the disease to be gone. Now we are into 'the space in between'. What are you going to fill the space with? Chemicals, surgery, drugs, or counselling? All of them? None of them? Now you are confused. Now you need to go into that space and just sit quietly and let the space be filled in your mind, with whatever best suits it.

The answer will come. Sigmund Freud says "When making a decision of minor importance, I have always found it advantageous to consider all the pros and cons. In vital matters, however, the decision should come from the unconscious, from somewhere within ourselves. In the important decisions of personal life, we should be governed by the deep inner needs of our nature." (Sigmund Freud)

When I died in 2009 I received brain damage that was severe. How did I heal my brain? I realized I have a problem and then I sat quietly and let the space in between give me the answer, or the energy. For me, I will then use Metatronic Energy to heal. You may use another energy that is different. I know that the solution to every problem is simple. It is the complications that we, as humans, place on a problem and the solution that stops us.

"The solution to every problem is simple. It is the space in between wherein the mystery lies."

That quote came from a book called *Skullduggery Pleasant* by Derek Landry. It was written for children aged 8 to 12-years-old and Skullduggery is a skeleton. I truly enjoy Landry's books and I read them often. I also find great peace in *'Artemis Fowl'* and *'Percy Jackson'* which are also children's books.

But perhaps my favourites, for wisdom, pleasure and anything else is absolutely anything by Christopher Brookmyre, a Scottish author. I love these books. They give me so much pleasure. I have learnt so much wisdom and gained so many insights from reading these books that I thoroughly recommend them to anyone.

You are far more likely to find me reading one of these books than sitting reading a 'new age' book, particularly as the teachings they so often recommend are not easily put into place in a real human life.

And you are, after all, here to be a human.

I don't have much time to meditate, or ring bells, or go off on a week-long retreat by myself. I thoroughly recommend you do this if you have the time, the money or the inclination. I have too many children and also too many roller coasters to ride to do that.

I am not telling you that you shouldn't. I am telling you that if you can't, this does not make you less spiritual than anybody else. In fact, in Heaven, when I went there last time, that is what I was told – your task is to be HUMAN, not SPIRIT. You are already 100% spirit. You already are. Now you need to learn to be human.

What makes people ill?

The one thing that has stood out 'in session' with people, above all else to me, is that those that are the most unwell are those people who are the most unhappy within themselves. They are discontent in their heart. The people who feel trapped, useless, unloved, angry, bitter or frustrated are far more likely to have a serious illness as a result of these feelings. People who felt they were living a life of duty or service – not because they wanted to – but because they felt that they had no choice were also likely to be ill as a result of the burdens of care. Even people who were really happy but harboured a secret desire to do more, be more, have more, were at risk of becoming ill. A person who is truly content with who they are and what they have is very unlikely to become ill.

If you are living for somebody else, you *are* dying for yourself.

We all have to do things that we don't really want to do. Trust me; I do, from time to time. I make the children's beds, I cook the dinner, I do the shopping and I stay home when I would much rather be out at Dreamworld, riding roller coasters. But I do all these things with the awareness of what this could do to me if I tried to deny it and I make sure that I fit in plenty of my time.

Before I realized what unrecognized resentment could do, I used to feel like the martyr. Then I realized that if I was going to do it, I had better get happy about that, or I had better stop doing it, no matter what the cost, because ultimately the cost would be serious illness.

I personally feel that illness is far worse than death. Imagine being trapped in a bed on a perfect summer day, a cool wind blowing across your face, the sound of the surf in your ears, and there you are stuck in bed, with cancer, or vertigo, or as a paraplegic.

But perhaps the more important question to ask is what makes a person be alive and yet dead inside, when they could live?

Fun. Love. Enjoyment. Pleasure. Satisfaction. Freedom. Choice.

All of these emotions are what you can choose to feel, even when you are in an untenable position. Truly. If you choose to take satisfaction, have pleasure and regard something unbearable as your *choice*, you will survive it. Viktor Frankl, who is the father of Psychotherapy, proved this, in the development of his therapy – therapy that he created in the soil of Auschwitz.

He realized, as a small Jewish person that the Germans could trammel his body, crush his mind, steal his clothes and torture him but that they could not tell him how to *feel*.

Fiona's case.

Hi Carmel, I have metastatic melanoma which is from four years ago. It originally started from a mole on my left bum cheek which I noticed started to bleed which was diagnosed with melanoma once removed.

Three years later I found a lump in my groin which was once again removed and diagnosed with melanoma again. To my shock I was then put in hospital and had all the lymph nodes removed in my left groin. On the pet scan it only showed three lymph nodes but when they came out there was five out of eight with cancer in them.

I was then told I had to go to Peter McCallum's, where I was asked to go in a trial for radiation therapy which had a 10% chance of it working. I chose not to do it as I have wanted to have a baby forever and just can't find the right man.

After six months I had to see my oncologist who I asked if I could have another scan because of wanting to have a baby. Anyway – bad news. She let me have a CT scan, which I had to wait another month for and bad news again. She said it was starting to spread. I have a 3 1/2cm tumor in my lower abdomen, three small lymph nodes about 1cm each in my stomach and one near my left shoulder.

You could imagine the shock I had and then to be told that it was very aggressive. I feel very well at the moment and I'm very athletic – just don't feel sick at all but have seen the cancer on the computer screen.

My oncologist told me that if we can't kill it or put it in remission I have two years to live.

This can't happen. I have too much living to do and I'm doing IVF mid March to save some eggs for myself.

Please if you can't help me that would be great.

My next scan is on the 12th of March.
Fiona

Some you win, some you lose.

This is one of the saddest and most heartbreaking cases I have ever worked on. Fiona came to see me because she had melanoma. Fiona was a lovely young lady who had first noticed a mole on her left bottom cheek. Upon investigation it was discovered that this was a melanoma. She was also now in a relationship with a man and she wanted her to have children with him.

It turned out that Fiona had trouble conceiving so they decided to continue on the IVF program Fiona had already started, but the treatment had created something in her body and the melanoma was now out of control. It was spreading fast and Fiona was sicker than she realized.

Fiona had issues with her mother and the way she had raised Fiona. The mere mention, the act and the thought of trying to have a baby had reignited the melanoma in Fiona, inspiring it to new, destructive levels. I could see that the cancer was now throughout her body, invading the bowels, inching up into the lungs and Fiona thought that she had it beat. I was just a check-up.

It had started with the mother and the family issues. Fiona deciding to have her own family had been an energetic flash fire for Fiona. And where it had started in her was where I would start with it.

The left side is the female/mother side. The bottom is ruled by the base chakra and the base chakra is family issues. The melanoma is a skin cancer; skin is also the base chakra. And cancer is anger, pure and simple. Therefore, Fiona had melanoma because she was angry over issues that related to her mother and having and raising children. This cancer was aggressive and would follow the path of anger in her body. All of it made sense. The bowels are family, tribal issues; the lungs hold the emotional issues and issues of love.

The trouble was – here was a beautiful, fit looking young woman sitting in front of me who was planning a life that she had dreamed of for years, with a new man.

And she was dying and she did not yet know that. Fiona had at best, from looking at her energy, six months to live. The IVF had drastically reduced her life span.

How do you tell a person who is determined to live that the very thing she is doing to live is killing her? How do you tell her that the relationship she was in and wanting to have children with her partner were killing her?

Fiona and I talked for a while and I laid pathways through her body, then I dropped the Metatronic Energy into her.

I asked her to go back to her oncologist and have some tests done, telling her that I was concerned the cancer was spreading into her bowels. I could feel and see the cancer in her bowels. Fiona acknowledged she had a fear about that, that she was feeling tired and it was harder for her to exercise.

We spoke about the need for her to use the energy I had put through her to let go of the issues that were destroying her body. Fiona promised to do her best and then she left.

Within a fortnight Fiona had emailed me to let me know that she had seen her oncologist and that he had confirmed she now had cancer in her bowels. Fiona was being placed in hospital and wondered if I would be able to come to hospital and give her some help.

When I got to the hospital later that week, I went straight to Fiona's room. She was lying in the bed waiting to go for her next treatment. I looked at her energy and I could see that she was not strong enough to face anymore chemotherapy. Also, because her immune system was so low, the cancer was still spreading. I talked to Fiona for a while, adjusted her energy and removed what harm I could from the drugs already used on her and so that the future chemo would be more effective.

This visit, Fiona also expressed concern about money and about being able to afford to live. She was not able to work right now due to the treatment, but she laughed about how much life insurance she had and how great it was that her doctor had agreed to write a letter, stating she had less than 12 months to live. This meant that the life insurance company would pay out 50% of her policy. Fiona had basically sealed her future. She would not have to have children that she thought she wanted but was afraid to have; she had enough money to live the rest of the time she had left. She would not have to resolve any issues with her family.

I thought back to the email she had sent me. She had finished off by saying –'Please if you *can't* help me that would be great.' I knew that Fiona was more afraid of living than of dying.

I finished the session and I left the hospital knowing that I would never see Fiona again.

Result: Fiona was dead within a month of that visit.

Some you win. Some you lose. That is the way of being a healer, whether you are a doctor, a Medical Intuitive or a facilitator, it is the same. Her doctor would have been as upset as I was. Her doctor would have tried his best, with best intent, with the only tools that he knew to use, and then having lost, he would have no doubt grieved.

You cannot save everybody, or even help everybody. The great unknown is the client themselves. You may know exactly what they need. You may give them what they need but it does not mean they will get well.

You are the great unknown in your life and you are the best person to chart the map that is you. Look at your life, the colours you wear, the food that you eat, the movies you watch, the books you read.

What are these things saying about you?
Is this the message you want to spread?
Are you living for you, or for other people?
Is your heart peaceful?

You know, it is not normal, or optimal, to be unhappy a lot of the time, or tired all the time, or angry all of the time. If you are any of these things, look within. It is *not* something that is being done *to* you by someone else. It is something you are doing to you by *choice*. I know that sometimes circumstances tell us that we are stuck. That has happened to me also. But if that is happening to you, choose to make it your choice. Or realize that when something happens again and again, it is a pattern.

You are not responsible for the way others treat you. You are responsible for the way that you respond to their treatment and for how you respond to how it makes you feel.

That is power.

Exercise:

To find out who, and where you are blaming other people for your life, and then to take back your power.

Spend a bit of time writing down where you are giving away your power so that you can reclaim your life.

Who are you blaming for the bad luck or misfortune in your life?

When All Else Fails

Who is responsible for your happiness?

Chapter Four:

The who and the why. A job description

Live out of your imagination, not your history.
- Stephen Covey

The first question to answer in this section is what does a Medical Intuitive actually do that a doctor or psychologist or clairvoyant does not do? Is this another superfluous profession, or something that might be useful to you?

A Medical Intuitive is actually like all three of those professions rolled into one person.

I describe myself as a human MRI scan who tells you *what* is going on, as well as *why* it is going on.

Most concisely people come to see me, sit in front of me and we talk. Then I tell them what I am seeing and we discuss it. Sometimes they know about what I am describing and sometimes they don't. Often people come to me because they know they are unwell, but they do not know why, what is wrong with them or how it will manifest. Often people come because they already know that they are sick and they want me to tell them how a treatment will succeed, or not, and also why – emotionally – they are sick.

A Medical Intuitive identifies the cause of your symptoms, both at the physical level and the emotional/spiritual levels. *Every* illness commences in the emotional/spiritual levels.

For instance, the cause/event may be something that happened to you when you were six years old and that you have forgotten about, or put aside as unimportant. Even though you have forgotten what happened, this event still set up a 'resonance' within you that sent out a signal to the Universe, telling the Universe that this sort of event was something you now expected, and that you could deal with. In essence, you begin to manifest events for your own comfort, even if it is not a comfortable event to you.

You may have been born into a family of people who were timid and did not stand up for themselves, gone to school to be bullied, grown up and married a person who was also a bully – emotional or physical – and then onto a job where the boss or co-workers were bullies. An unfortunate series of events that you can halt, if you wish to.

But before you can alter it, you need to acknowledge that you are the one who allowed it. You are *not* the one who did it, created it, asked for it or are responsible for it. But you are the one who allowed it. It is my job, a Medical Intuitives job, to point that out to you.

Many of us have met someone who always seems to have partners who play around on them. No matter how many partners they have, or how different these new people look and behave, in the end, the relationship goes the same way. Some people just always lose things, or lose jobs, or crash cars, or gamble everything away. They break bones, get robbed, get assaulted and more. The most incredible litany of bad luck seems to follow some people around. Just as incredibly good luck, the 'luck of the Irish' seems to follow other people around. The people who have this terrible luck will tell you that they don't like it – and they don't, but they do expect it, they do know how to deal with it and they are braced for it.

A Medical Intuitive will read your energy system to uncover these resonances in you and to link these resonances or blocks for you to the actual, or the possible, illnesses that are happening in your body. They can look at what *will* also happen in the future and then help you to stop it happening. I know that I will see illnesses up to seven years in the future, as a possible event. My aim is not to tell you about what may happen in seven years time, but to use this skill cleverly enough that I can see it and start removing it from you before you need to develop it. If you can maintain the change I help you to effect, we will be successful. I will tell you what you are at risk of developing, though.

How do I do this? I will do this by watching mentally the progress of your body, if you continue to do as you are doing. It is through the use of forward seeing. All illnesses start as a block caused by a resonance signal in the energy system. A Medical Intuitive is an early warning system.

If you *already* have an illness then a Medical Intuitive is there to tell you what you can do to potentially reverse your condition. There may be no reversal.

I will look at someone's energy system and I will see what they are missing in terms of vitamins, minerals, amino's or exercise. I will also see if they are taking something that is toxic to them and I can see if a course of treatment will be as successful as they hope it will be.

When All Else Fails

Sometimes people get sick and die, just as I did. There really was nothing wrong with me *physically* and there still isn't. My heart just stopped for no reason that could be found and for no reason that the medical profession could see other than my heart was emotionally too heavy to continue.

I knew I was going to die, but I was so comfortable with all the things that were causing my death that I could not work out how to let them go to change this before it happened.

But I knew, when I returned, that if I did not alter how I was feeling, I would quickly die again. I wanted to live for a while longer. I am not afraid of dying. I am not afraid of death, but it is different to be with someone and be dead, than to be alive and be there with them on Earth. The ability to hold their hand and feel the warmth is very nice and I wanted to live with my husband and my children.

I needed to know what I did and did not do that allowed me to die.

Medicine could not answer my questions. So I went on the journey to discover. I asked what, why, how and who.

We are none of us finished. If we are alive there is something more for us to learn or do. Even a Medical Intuitive is a work in progress.

Carmel Bell

What is it like, inside a session?

A brief description of setting up a session.

When you come to see me, the first thing you will notice is that my room is a little like a lounge room, with comfortable armchairs to sit on and nice pictures on the wall, but up high and out of the way. The lighting is dim and there is water to drink. I also make sure that there are paper and pens in there for you to take notes of anything we may discuss. There is very little in there to distract me. The walls are a light, plain colour, which makes it all the better to see your energy.

We sit opposite each other and talk. I have set questions that I will ask because I am looking for hooks in your energy body, or a loss of resonance. These are questions I have worked out over the years that are like reflex actions in everybody's energy field. Everybody, when asked about their mother will have an optimum response. A different response will indicate a problem, or a 'hook'.

Once I find the hooks I will know where to start looking in you and I will know what kind of issues you are developing. It is so simple and so clean that it is beautiful. It will take me only a few minutes to know what I need to know, then you and I need to talk about it so that you can accept and assume responsibility for it. If you do not take ownership you will never heal.

I draw your attention to an issue, you assume responsibility for how you feel and your part, if any, in the event(s) and then we work out an action plan to remove it.

This action plan may include treatment options for you, such as tests you may request your doctor to perform, or herbs you will need to ask your naturopath to dispense, or homoeopathics you may need to see a homeopath about, or relationships that you may need to consider. Because I am a dedicated Medical Intuitive, I do not do any of these other things. I am not trained in any other modality, so I have no bias or leaning towards one over another.

After we have talked, I will use Metatronic Energy to start a balance in your energy system and then I will teach you how to manage the flow of this energy yourself so that you get maximum benefit. I will also teach you how to deal with anything that arises from the healing.

The Rower

"Your lower back is very painful and you feel that you cannot live like this any longer." I looked at the man sitting in front of me: in his 50's, attractive, fit looking, healthy enough in his body. He was a man who loved to row, but now pain was holding him back. "Every time you row, you hurt. It hurts to sit, to lie down, to move." Doing what he loved was painful. Interesting.

He nodded, "Yes, that's right. I've tried everything I can think of but I can't find the problem." He looked at me expectantly. There was no challenge in his gaze. He had been referred to me by his doctor who was also a client of mine and who respected the work I do. I looked at the notes I had written whilst I had been talking to him, noting the energy swirls I had drawn, and where, on the diagram of the body that I had before me, I had drawn them. During a session I sit and draw absently whilst listening or speaking and this drawing would become part of my record of an energy system at the time of our consultation.

Although the energy system changes continuously, this drawing was the best way to record the most pertinent points for memory purposes. "Let's talk about how you feel constantly under the hammer. You are disconnected from your family, your father in particular. You feel nothing you have done has been good enough. How hard do you have to try?" I asked him. "The real problem is the anxiety that you suffer from. The anxiety that cripples you and stops you from achieving the things you want to achieve."

David started to cry, softly, and it seemed unnoticed by him, the tears flowed down his face. "Your back pain now is just another way to stop you doing the things you want to do. This is your way of punishing yourself."

"I know..." he sighed. I shook my head. David's body was reacting to a lifetime of stress, a lifetime of trying to be what his family wanted him to be, rather than what he needed to be. A lifetime held in every cell of his body that had led to a sore lower back, high anxiety levels and a general malaise in his life. David had a wife that he loved and children who were all well, and achieving in their lives. From the outside looking in, it looked like David had it all and perhaps he did. He had everything but self belief – the ability to achieve the goals that he had set. Anxiety sounds like a small issue, but it is crippling. And back pain each time you performed something you loved to do was also crippling.

The real problem was David. He was not who, or what, he wanted to be. He was living for other people and that meant he was dying for himself. No matter what he did, he could not seem to find the approval that he sought. The sadness was that even if his parents were proud of him, and did love him, David could not 'feel' it. He would hear and see only what he expected.

Constantly trying to fill other people's expectations had left almost no room for his own peace of mind.

David and I talked about what was happening in his life, how it had made him unwell and uncomfortable and how he could be healthier than before.

"David, I am going to use a technique that I have developed to unblock the energy that you have stored in your body and has made you ill. I use an energy called Metatronic Energy and I am also going to teach you how to manage the energy that I put through you so that you can achieve maximum results. Okay?"

David nodded. "Okay." I indicated to a small stool in between us.

"Could you please sit here," I asked. David stood up from the chair he was on, walked to the stool and sat down. I stood behind him and called Metatronic Energy. I could feel the light tingling of Metatronic Energy on the palm of my right hand, bouncing there, waiting to be told what to do. By calling this energy onto my right hand, I made sure that it did not first enter through my body and then into David. David would receive the full benefit of pure, unadulterated energy, rather than something that has passed through a conduit.

Calmly I dropped the energy into the top of David's head so that it flowed down into his crown chakra. As it flowed off my hand and into David I asked Metatron to release the unnecessary stories from David's body. Then I turned my attention to making sure that I could feel the energy as it passed through each chakra. Once I could feel energy flowing through his entire system, I recharged David with Bio Energy and then I stood back. I did nothing more. All this took only a few minutes for me to do. Metatronic Energy is intelligent and interactive and hardly takes any thought, once you have laid the 'pathways'. Metatronic Energy will keep working long after I have stopped channelling it into a person's body.

The most time consuming part of a session is getting people to understand and accept responsibility for their own health. It is getting people to let go of all the stories they have told themselves throughout their life. "I could give up smoking, except I am so angry." Or "I would be a success if only someone believed in me." In most people the story has become more important than happiness or health.

We all have free will, we make choices for ourselves and because of this, your choice, I make no guarantees of any outcome from any healing; I cannot know what will get healed because so much depends on what you are willing to let go of. But I can tell you that you will leave a session with a greater sense of peace – and usually – determination.

"I can feel that!" David exclaimed. I smiled.

'I hope so." I replied. I finished off the session by explaining to David why he needed to care for his system and how. I talked to him about how he could release the unwanted information that would arise as a result of this energy work. How if he held this unwanted information in him, it would make him unwell again.

I am not in control as to what will be revealed or released as the outcome from the energy work, but as David's ill health was mostly caused by the issues lodged in his base chakra, it was quite likely that he would remember many things that had occurred to him in childhood. These recollections would be both 'good and bad' recollections. There really is no value judgement on them from me – it is just that most people prefer to remember the happy and suppress the sad, but both types of memories go into the chakras and clog them up. You need to remove the energy from both if you wish to be energetically free.

David was likely to find, over the next few weeks, that he would remember many childhood stories and that his parents or siblings would contact him somehow. All of these happenings would allow David the opportunity to dump issues from his chakras and reframe how he interacts with his family. As a result of this interaction, he would find that his ill health would decrease or disappear.

David left our session, smiling and hopeful. He had had a shift in his awareness and, although his ill health was not life-threatening, it was life crippling but now he would be able to heal and improve the quality of his life. Even if his illness had been life-threatening, he would have the tools to turn it around.

Research in the past has shown that all spontaneous cures of cancer were preceded by a dramatic shift in awareness. The force responsible for healing lies within each of us, not in the doctor or alternative healer, or a pill you take. But You. Inside of You. In the *decision* to take the pill, to see the healer, to go to the doctor or to let go of the story you have clung to for so long. To heal you need to accept full responsibility for every moment of every day of your life. You cannot give away your responsibility to anyone. You cannot blame anyone for your feelings. Ever. Some people find that overwhelming, so used have we become to 'victim' mentality – to finding someone to blame for the things that happen to us. But that is the way to lose power. You cannot take on another person's responsibility. If someone has hurt you, that is their guilt to bear. And you cannot ask them to assume responsibility for what you do with the experience you gained. You cannot ask them to assume responsibility for you ruining your life anymore than you can ask them to take the credit for your successes as a result. You are responsible for you and you alone.

Every moment matters. How you deal with each moment matters. You being consciously awake, as far as possible, in each moment, matters. You living a life full of awareness, integrity and courage is essential.

Often people ask me why I am asking them about something I can see in their energy field in a session when I talk to them about their health. They do not realize how important every thought, moment, belief, is. They want to believe that their feelings towards other people have not had anything to do with where they are today. They want to believe that the anger they carry for slights against them could not have caused the cancer that now resides in their body. They also want to believe that hurts they have suffered when they were a child or any age, could not be affecting them now. That if they have gone through years of therapy that they should be 'healed'. So many people I see bear enormous guilt because they feel they have somehow 'failed' to get well. They have talked their problems over, many times, and yet they still feel terrible. And yet, the same things keep happening to them. What these people have not realized is that all the moments are residing in their cells. We need to release these moments from the cells. If these moments stay trapped inside the cells, they send out an energy signal attracting to you similar situations. You may not like the situation, but you know how to deal with it. Even though it is often destructive if the signal is based on negative events, this is also a self preservation technique. At least you don't have to think too hard about how to react and behave.

I teach people to self heal by releasing these moments from their cells, their bodies, so that they can get about the business of living the life that they wanted to live.

Other people want to see me and have me 'heal' them. The majority of people leave my room healthier than they came in, but some people do leave in tears when I explain that now they will have to let go of the very thing that has fuelled their life for years. Issues they think could not possibly be linked to their health and happiness they suddenly discover have been killing them and now they have to let them go. For instance ... they have to throw out the anger at their parents, perhaps, for not giving them the support they needed to become the artist, or anything else, they wanted to be. An anger that is so subtle and so old, they do not even realize it exists. To you, standing on the outside, this may sound easy, but it is a very hard task, because of its subtle nature, this anger may have shaped so many aspects of the person's life that it has created who they are and how they see themselves.

Who are you when you are no longer the person you thought you were?

This is a question that all of us have to face. None of us are exempt from that journey. A lot of people, who don't heal, won't answer that question. They want to believe that someone else is responsible. This is a belief that will keep them trapped and disempowered. They give their power over to someone else – their parents, their doctor, their psychologist, their partner. No-one else should make your choices for you .They can help you to make a choice, but you must accept responsibility for the ultimate choice, and end result.

David was struggling because he believed his life was decided for him by other people and when he did what he wanted to do, it felt like he was doing the wrong thing, thus it would cause him pain, both physically and emotionally. The only way for him to feel better was to realize that. Once he did that, he could decide to be happy where he was, or change it. As an aside, David is now happy.

You cannot change anything that has happened to you, but you *can* change how you feel about it.

Result: David feels that the results that he gained from our sessions are more profound and more dramatic than anything else he has tried before. He is a much more content and confident man than he was. He reports that he feels much healthier and sure of himself. Life has improved a lot for David. He is able to row, pain free now. He continues to ground, seal and dump.

Overburdened by responsibility

I looked at the man as he hobbled through my door. Middle aged, bent, twisted, quite unstable on his feet despite two walking sticks. I knew that he frequently used a wheelchair because he had asked my assistant about wheel chair access over the phone.

"Hello," I started, "I'm Carmel Bell,"

"Uh," he grunted in a disinterested way. "Neville."

"Can you sit here, please, Neville?" I asked him, indicating the chair slightly to the left of him. Neville moved laboriously to the chair and carefully manipulated his body until he could sit.

It was obvious that Neville lived in a lot of pain. Every day was a challenge to move around his environment. His face reflected that challenge; closed off, darkened and unwell looking.

As I often did, I wondered what had bought Neville to see me. I asked.

"Who referred you to me?"

Neville was looking around the room, at anything but me. "Susanne."

I really wasn't sure which Susanne, but I sent a silent nod to her in thanks, then I began.

Neville sat in a chair in front of me at an ideal distance away so that I can see his energy field whilst we spoke. I just talked. There was no particular rhyme or reason as to what questions I chose to ask, I just followed my intuition beyond the first few questions. There are a few very important standard questions that I do ask about their family history. Every one of us is a construct of our family. You cannot escape them, even in Heaven.

And on earth it is often worse. We call this field Epigenetics and it is a fascinating study of your ancestor's effects on your body now.

"Is your father alive?" I began with my first question.

"Yes, he is." Neville answered me as I watched his energy field closely.

Neville had severe scoliosis of the spine. He was angry and unhappy. He was also, trapped beneath this, an extremely loving, caring, generous man who has lived with pain and discomfort for many years.

Neville started out happy in life, but it soon turned out to be something he did not want. He was the eldest son of two dependant parents. He had siblings, but neither his brother nor sister wanted the responsibility for the parents, so Neville ended up in the family business rather than becoming what he wanted to be.

His brother and sister both married and left home to live their lives, leaving Neville to carry the load.

At 30, Neville had been tall and vigorous. By the time he was 45; he was bent over and twisted from a spine that was warping rapidly. He was still single and he was even less happy than he had been before.

Then by the time he was 50, Neville was very sick. His spine was twisted badly and he had a metal rod which had been surgically inserted to keep him upright. He was hardly able to walk; in pain throughout most of his body and angry about his life. He exuded anger. If you were anywhere near Neville, you had to feel it.

Neville was blaming anybody but himself for his life. It was easy to see why. He had spent his life trying to do the 'right thing' and it is never easy to say to someone who you care about, "Bad luck, you are on your own." But that is part of the cycle of life. Your parents gave birth to you, but they do not own you.

There is a balance between being sacrificial and being helpful. You can find other ways around most problems.

Neville should have recognized that he needed his own life and perhaps he could have helped his father find a member of staff to work in the business whilst Neville went to university.

Perhaps he would have then met a woman and had his own family. Instead he came to me, angry and bitter.

Result: After a few sessions of releasing the stories and teaching Neville how to deal with his energy, he went on, despite his age, to form a relationship with a woman and to learn a healing modality himself. Neville became one of the loveliest, happiest and gentle men I know.

His parents live on.

The point is, this is your life. You and you alone have control over that life and what you do with it. Even if you are imprisoned, you have control. No one can control the way you feel. They can torture you, torment you, make you dance, insult you, but they cannot get inside your mind and make you feel or think. And if you die, then you are free again, too.

The third client

My third client for the day was a man who had told me that he was a practitioner of a small and unusual Buddhist sect that did not believe in people having sex. He was quite adamant about this. His partner was also a client of mine and she had told me the same thing. This couple had been together for five years but had not once had sex with each other.

The problem was that Frank was depressed and anxious. His work was suffering and he no longer found any joy in his life, yet he did not want to end his relationship. According to Frank, if he could just stop feeling so miserable, he would be happy.

He had come to see me so that he would be find happiness.

There was not a lot that I could do for Frank. My heart went out to him in complete compassion.

"Don't you miss sex?" I asked.

"Yes, I do. But I have learnt to do without it."

"Was that your choice?"

"Well, not really," he admitted, 'It was Mandy's choice'." I looked at him silently. "She doesn't really like sex." I remained silent.

"She was hurt once … " He explained, shrugging.

"So now you live together but you don't sleep together. How is work going?" I asked him.

"Badly." Frank shook his head. "I just don't feel any happiness when I am there anymore." Frank was a psychotherapist and did have a busy practice.

We talked for a little longer, about his growing lethargy, lack of joy and bouts of aggression that he was feeling. I explained to him that if he stayed in a relationship that did not serve him, he would continue to ail. It is not natural for a human to forego sex and then to live in an intimate relationship with a sexual partner who was not a sexual partner. Frank's body and spirit were both receiving mixed signals.

On closer discussion it was revealed that Frank had been raised by a very strict religious family who did not believe that nice people had sex. His whole life had been full of confused messages about the value of fun and the healthy pleasures of the body.

I ran Metatronic Energy through Frank and he left, happier than when he arrived.

There is nothing wrong with sex between two consenting adults. In fact, it is probably the most fun you can have legally, without harm. No part of the body is dirty, or lacking in sacredness, or something to be ashamed of. But when sex or something involved with sex is used to overpower, hurt or maim another person, then it *is* wrong.

The two things we cannot do in Heaven and that we can do on Earth is having sex and eating food. We came to be in human form in part so that we could enjoy ourselves by having sex. Yet we have so many problems with sex. We hurt each other and betray each other using sex. This beautiful and pleasurable and free act is turned into a mockery.

How do you feel about sex? Are you happy with your attitude? Do you allow your body to feel beautiful and sensual and desirable? Or do you choose to feel dirty, have sex with the lights out? Refuse to laugh about it, talk about it?

If you are low in energy, one of the most invigorating and refreshing acts you can perform is to have sex.

But like most good things, this is open to abuse and sadly there are lots of humans who will feel free to use it for abuse. They rape other people, mutilate them through circumcision, behave sexually with children, have sex with animals or deny their partner the right to a free and healthy sex life.

You are free to choose for yourself to have sex or not, but you are not free to choose for your partner, if you are in a relationship.

Result: Frank's relationship lasted a few months more, and then ended naturally. He is now happily re-partnered and his own practice is thriving.

Anger

Client: female age 55 – high cholesterol issues.

Cheryl came to see me because her cholesterol was very high and she did not want to go on medication. I could see that her heart was being adversely affected by her health which was more worrying than the cholesterol. We began a history.

She had three children, one of whom was still too young to leave, her blood pressure looked high – which Cheryl confirmed. She told me that her ECG was normal, but I could see the lack of joy in her. When we kept talking she admitted she did not like her life but she did not know how to change it. She loved her husband but did not know how to get him to have more fun with her and she felt like she was just marking time. Her doctor wanted her on medicine and in counselling. Both were good suggestions, but really all they would do would be to get her to accept what she felt she could not change.

I knew Cheryl would have a heart attack if she did not make some choices. She wanted me to tell her what to do, or get her to be happy enough with what she had so that she would not mind what she did not have.

I couldn't. I asked her to take medication, I asked her to do some more exercise and I asked her to have some fun.

"Who with?" she almost cried. "There is no-one!" Which was the real point. Cheryl did not feel as if she belonged anywhere anymore and she felt that she was out of touch with all her friends. If Frank did not want to spend time with her, she was stuck.

I told her the consequences of continuing on as she was and although she was not happy about it, she accepted it.

After our session and healing, Cheryl went home. But Cheryl stayed in my mind because it did not feel like I achieved what I wanted to.

Three months later I received an email from her in response to an enquiry from me.

Carmel – thank you for your help. I thought that I would let you know that I had a small heart attack, as you were concerned about, but it is okay. Because of this, Frank and I have decided to take a holiday and leave the children to care for themselves while we are away. (of course we will take Bekky)
I am having fun. Thanks for the reminder.
Warm regards, Cheryl

Sometimes a poor result is a good result.

Finding patterns

I've shown four sessions in one day. Each of these people shared things in common, although you may not immediately see the commonality. They were all angry and disillusioned and doing something they did not really want to do.

But far more importantly, all of these people thought someone else was responsible for them being miserable and for them being happy, which is equally as burdensome for all involved.

Yet each one of them ended up in a different place, with a different illness. The reason for that is because of the different issues they were dealing with. Because of the difference, different chakras were being used to store the issues in.

To locate what chakra is the main issue in your life, you can look at either the different illnesses or what they mean, or at the different issues. For instance, issues to do with the family go into the base and issues about your lover go into the sacral. I recommend that you read Annette Hayes' book, or Louise Hayes' book. There are several really excellent books that will give you illnesses, causes, thoughts you can change for you to study.

When I am in a session, I like to know that I have in my mind all the knowledge that I need. Just as I keep in my mind the different body systems, I also keep in there the different chakras and what each one means. I have with me, inside me, the basic patterns that I really need to know and understand, such as the knowledge that if it is a skeletal problem, it is held in the base chakra and the base chakra deals with family problems, therefore let us focus on family if you have osteoporosis. Family can also mean work clusters, friend clusters, golf partners, and more. Any basic group that you hang out with or rely on can affect the base chakra.

But nobody has only one chakra in play – everybody has the heart chakra involved, regardless of everything else. Most people have the sacral and the solar because of their functions. I think that this only leaves the throat and the third eye and the crown out of play so far.

Who doesn't want to communicate their frustration at having an issue, talking to people around then and possibly also talking to the Divine? Meanwhile, your thoughts are firmly focused on what is happening. That covers the throat, the third eye and the crown chakras.

Suddenly the whole system is in a mess. If you start looking at what each chakra could mean and then each illness could mean you would be there for hours, going nuts.

What you need to do is focus on the *main* chakra that is a problem and then consider all the secondary chakras after that. Treat them all.

This is why I use Metatronic Energy and treat the whole system. This is why I talk to people and get the energy to map out a pathway through that person, without regard for my thoughts on the matter. Talking to a person about what is going on and talking about the causes of the issue will 'wake up' the whole energy system and put in pathways that you can use to clear the issue. I am creating a map through their body.

Every journey is the destination and it is also the road that led to the destination.

So remember that when you are ill, it is you, your *whole body*, not just one little bit that is ill. There are plenty of books that will tell you what each illness means individually and what mantra you should use to treat it. But let me caution you. You need to understand the systems and illnesses but without letting them box you in, or you may miss the real cause. If you miss the cause you will end up chasing the same problem around your body in 10 different disguises.

Also, look for patterns. On occasion the patterns are obvious, but what the patterns *signify* is not always quite so obvious. I have had days when everybody was born on the same birthday and that is sometimes five people born on July 24th, for instance. Other days, everybody had the same first name and I end up with a stream of people called Sally – silly things like that. I laugh, but I also think to myself – why? What is the *message* or the pattern? Life will always find a way to bring sense and a pattern to everything. Even snowflakes are beautifully patterned pieces of geometry.

Sometimes the connection is obvious straight away. All these people may have mother issues, or maybe their fathers all died when they were children. Perhaps they all work in the same sort of job, or grew up in the same town, or follow the same religion. The Universe is neat and organized and if you just sit back and wait, the organization will be shown to you.

You take what you have learnt each day, you go home and you allow the Universe to tell you what they mean by this. Doing this has allowed me to see and learn many things. I am able to take a block of people who have something in common and work out what the connecting thread is and what that means. Then the next time someone crosses my path with that thread, I am able to tell them what is likely to eventuate for them. Better still, I am also able to help them to stop it before it begins.

There are patterns in everything and everywhere. Nothing is accidental, every moment matters. Even music creates patterns in sand and water.

Exercise:

Start to think about your day, at the end of each day. Give yourself a few minutes of quiet time to see if you can spot a pattern that may be part of the reason why you are not as content as you would like to be.

Chapter Five:

The blocks to healing

Conflict cannot survive without your participation.
- Wayne Dyer

The blocks to healing

There are several blocks to healing. You may be surprised to learn that some people, possibly even you yourself, don't actually want to be well. It is not that you want to be sick, but the fact that you are sick gives you a cost benefit. The cost of being sick purchases you something else. Also, being well carries a particular burden. You need to be more responsible when you are well.

These are some of the benefits that people have told me that they have received over the years from being unwell.

Block One: Suffering from Over-Attention

It may be that you are receiving attention from being ill. This attention may be help with doing things like housework, or it may be people showing you that they love you.

It could be a partner staying with you, rather than leaving. It is remarkably common to hear of a marriage that was about to end when one of the partners became critically ill. And how you can leave when your wife or husband is on death's door? If you do, how many people are going to look at you and judge you to be the worst kind of horrible in the world? So you stay and they receive attention. Or they stay and you receive the love you rely on. What happens when you get well? Often they leave anyway. Of course, sometimes they stay – the time together may have been enough to renew your regard for one another. But how many times have you seen a person quickly re-partner after their partner has died? I have seen marriages take place within weeks.

Any attention you receive, that you would not have received when you were well is something that is a two-edged sword. We need it, but its very kindness can keep us crippled.

Block Two: Abundance

It may be financial support offered because you are sick or childcare given because you are too tired to do for yourself. Gardening, housework, shopping runs and a multitude of other benefits are often handed to us when we are in need. Thank the Universe that all of these things do come to us when we need them, but the caveat is that we need to become astute at realising when the benefit from receiving these things is less than the benefit from being well enough to do for ourselves. If you break your leg and use a wheelchair to get around without ever bothering to exercise, you may find that your leg becomes too weak to be used at all, long after the break has healed. You will be crippled by the kindness of the wheelchair.

I am definitely *not* telling you that you should not receive help. Of course you should. But you want to make sure that you also grow past the need for that help.

In the end, all these benefits, such as the housework are useful to the person receiving them. If they were to get well and stop receiving them, but are now so used to receiving them that they are crippled, how would they be able to function? So they choose to stay ill because they are afraid to *not be ill*.

The two-edged sword also tells us that there are people out there who are addicted to helping and therefore it is hard for that person/addict to help others become independent. Everything needs to be in balance.

If it is you who is unwell you may be scared of healing, or of being healed. You may be quite comfortable in your discomfort. You may even wonder –if you heal, what would be left of you? I understand that and I respect that. I want you to know what no matter what your illness happens to be, you can recover from it, whether you're 15, 50 or 100 and whether your illness is emotional or physical, if you *want to* recover. You don't have to recover and you are not a failure if you don't recover, but I urge you, if you think that this could be a factor in your lack of healing, look for it, find it, get rid of it and get well.

Block Three: Not bored enough

The fastest, most guaranteed way to get well is to get *bored* with being unwell.

I know that I really do not do 'unwell' very well. I hate lying in bed on a beautiful day when others are out playing. If it is raining, I want to jump in puddles. If it is sunny, I want to lie around and bask. If I see a travel ad, I immediately hanker to buy a ticket and go away. If there is a movie on, I want to watch it.

My attitude is that I want to suck the marrow out of life. I want to do everything, go everywhere and experience everything. Anytime I get sick, it gets in my way. I hate talking about it, living it, feeling it, breathing it. I have absolutely no time for it in me *at all.* And because of that attitude I have recovered from many illnesses.

Block Four: Guilt

What if you live in a family that has a genetic condition like diabetes, and you don't develop diabetes, but all the others do. You suffer from guilt.

What if you have a baby and your baby lives, but your sister who was also having a baby loses hers. Guilt.

What if you are faced with success and you come from a family that is full of failures. Guilt.

Your parents are alcoholics and you aren't? Guilt.

Siblings who are all fat and you are thin. Guilt.

The list is endless. You change the predicted path of your life and you will often be plagued with guilt. Many people unfortunately find this too hard to deal with. Many people cannot stand being more successful than their parents. When they are, they fall back onto guilt and they sabotage themselves.

They become what their family is or they leave the family.

Are you a saboteur?

Block Five: Forgetting to laugh.

Don't forget to laugh. You are funny. You are clever and amusing. Think of the fantastic game that you have been playing. Because you are funny and you are playing a game. You designed this; even if you don't want to believe that you did, you did.

How clever are you?

Imagine believing that every man is a bastard, because your father was an ignorant drunk who never cared and then, despite all your best attempts you end up with a husband who is an alcoholic. How funny is that? I mean, not funny, like in loony toons funny, but funny just the same, which is why all good comedies are based on absolute disasters. You can make a disaster out of a situation or you can make a joke. I admit that there are some things that I cannot laugh at, some tragedies that are too big, too heart wrenching, but there are not that many of them. The Second World War, not funny, September 11, not amusing at all.

But – sailing through the Atlantic, right into an iceberg, the only one there, within miles, in an unsinkable ship and sinking it! What? What was all that about?

If you don't laugh, you cry, and you know, crying is exhausting and draining. If you have something happen to you that you cannot change, alter or otherwise fix up, you may as well work at seeing something funny in it.

I promise you that every single person I have seen heal against impossible odds, including myself, did so with laughter as their boon companion and every single person that I have seen die did so with grief about their life, blaming someone else, giving their power away to the person or persons or drugs that has 'killed' them.

Laugh.

There are many more blocks to healing that you may need to nut out and think about for yourself but these are the main ones. I encourage you to look at what is stopping you from having the life you want. What is your block?

Many people will tell you that it is fear of failure, but I promise you that I have seen fear of success be far more destructive.

I would like you to think about your life and what you are gaining out of being where you are, if anything. You may not be gaining anything at all and that is usually good. But if you are ill and you are gaining from that, then you may want to consider what it is really costing you.

Some people definitely need all the help that they can get so that they can live, get well again if they can, or be supported. But if you are getting more from your illness than you want to admit to, think about it and then go out and live.

Block Six: The way you think

What? The way I think?

Yes. The way you think. Your thoughts are responsible for the way you feel and the way you respond to every situation.

No-one can control the way you think except you. Even when someone is talking to you, you can be standing there saying anything you like to yourself. You can be imitating them, mocking them and agreeing with them. And all this in private and all in silence.

The single biggest block to your healing is the way you think.

The single biggest creator of your illness is the way you think.

What we are going to do in this book is give you an option. This option is the ability to choose to think another way.

Every situation can be viewed from a different angle. What is your angle? How do you like to see things? Are you a glass half full or glass half empty person?

What assumptions are you making about your life, your interactions, your future. When you assume, you make an ass out of you and me.

Exercise:

What is *your* block to healing?
    What are you receiving from your illness that may be keeping you ill?
    What are you gaining from your situation in life?
    How would your life look if you were not ill or unhappy?

All of these blocks can be dealt with later on when you learn how to use Metatronic Energy, if you have recognized that you have the block.
    Know yourself.

Chapter Six:

Finding out why

Change will not come if we wait for some other person or some other time. We are the ones we've been waiting for. We are the change that we seek. - **Barack Obama**

Perhaps the real difficulty is in finding out *why* you have not become well. I promise you that the body wants to be healthy. The desire inside every cell is to be well. The desire is to be healthy and happy. No being, no cells want to be sick, depressed or die before their time. Not one single bit of you wants that, except for you. Your mind, your psyche will choose to be sick and will choose to die. If you don't want to yet, you need to find out *why*.

Next you will have to be prepared to go into what I call the 'Heart of Darkness'. You know, that place isn't so hard, or so bad and it can actually be quite a lot of fun. We are often raised in this world to *not* be self aware and to feel that if we spend a lot of time on true self exploration that we are being selfish and bad. True self exploration involves understanding what darkness we *can* commit. Most people *could* commit horrible crimes, if given the right incentive and the right tools. What makes us truly marvellous is not that we would not do this, but that we could do this and we *choose not to*. Your choice is you. You are defined by your choices. To deny that we could be mean, nasty, and petty is to give that dark side of our nature power, the power to sneak up on us and hit us with a 2 x 4 piece of wood. I agree that there is nothing quite as boring as a narcissist, but there is nothing wrong and plenty that is right in looking at yourself and understanding you and your journey and of seeing into your 'Heart of Darkness'.

We are told that when we go into the heart, we should wallow. The thing is, you need to look, but you don't need to dwell. Go in; roll around for a while, but then, for heaven's sake! Get out whilst you can! You are here to live, right here, right now. Even when it is rotten, crappy, awful, lousy, live, have fun and laugh.

Let me be clear about this, though. You can spend a lot of time talking about your life, your problems, what is wrong with you, how miserable you are and generally how unfair it has all been without getting any results, There are plenty of people who use counselling and therapy as a means to stay stuck, going over and over and over the same old issues again and again, crying, weeping, moaning and getting sick. They are doing the same old thing again and again. This is not going inside. This is not being self aware. This is not progress. This is not healing, or any form of positive. This is another form of addiction, harder to break than heroin and far more destructive.

There comes a time when you have to say 'Enough! No more wallowing. I am done with this.' And more sternly to yourself, 'Heal.'

Insights

If the same things are happening in your life, ask yourself what the one common denominator might be? You. You are the common denominator.

If you always have relationships that fail and have partners who abuse you, either physically or emotionally, then ask yourself why? What is it in you that attracts these people to you and you to them? No-one else is choosing them, or making you be involved. These people may come from completely different backgrounds from each other, which can make identification of the pattern tricky unless you are self aware. Stand back, look honestly at yourself and your situation and save yourself some grief.

If you *own* your situation and what has happened to you, no matter how horrid that might feel at first, you will actually be able to use Metatronic Energy to get 'rid' of whatever 'it' is.

If you were attacked, for instance, and you acknowledge that this may have happened because you were at that place and at that time this happened to you, you *can* let it go. This does *not* in any way let the attacker off the hook, at all. Nor does it make you responsible for the actions of another person. But it does give you the ability to move out of victim, to move out of anger and fear, to move out of all the other destructive patterns that you can set up and to throw away the harm done to you. Assuming your own responsibility gives you back your power. It means you can do something about your situation and be powerful and in control once more.

When I decided to move out of home I purchased a rug and some stools for my new and as yet unknown home. I was excited about my purchase. I trotted them home and proudly showed my father who thoughtfully burst my bubble by saying to me. "Great. Now wherever you go you will need a truck."

"Huh?" I said.

"Before you bought these you were free to go wherever you wanted and now you need a truck to move you. Congratulations."

He was right. But the beauty was, because I owned these things I could get rid of them. I was not given them; I purchased them with my own money. So I was free to throw them away. I was not minding them for someone else. They were mine.

Same as if someone hurts me. Their words and actions are theirs and they have to own them. My thoughts and feelings and responses in response to them are mine and I can change them because they are mine. Make me angry, I can stop being angry. Make me sad, I can stop being sad. Hurt me and I can choose not to hurt you back.

Powerful. That is what that ability to not react unless I choose to, makes me.

Client: Female aged 49 – single mother 2 children. Pensioner. Manic depression. Nerve damage to the neck – Accountant.

Mary was the saddest woman you would ever hope to meet. She came in dragging her feet, reeking of cigarette smoke, bedraggled and looking a wreck. It was easy to see that she had been an attractive woman once, but not anymore.

She had manic depression, she was a single mother with two children and yet another failed relationship as she had just left her partner because he was abusive, Mary said.

I could see that Mary was a very smart woman and beneath the dishevelled exterior, she had a bright future, if she wished to.

When I looked at her energy system as we talked I could see that Mary was incredibly angry. She was not settled in herself and she hated men. She thought that everyone and everything owed her a living. She had been married twice, both marriages had ended. She had then swung between being a lesbian and being heterosexual. She lived on a pension even though she was a qualified accountant. She did not work. She could not see the point.

So what was wrong? Why could Mary not snap out of this and live a life?

Mary was angry over *possibly* being abused when she was three. One of her cousins had abused her, she thought. She could not even be sure because it was a 'reclaimed' memory from a counselling session and what I could see was that she did not want to know the truth, and it really did not matter anyway. Why ruin your life and if you were abused, give the abuser the rest of your life as payment?

Mary walked away feeling happy but in reality, no better and never likely to be.

One of the hardest parts of being a healer, from any profession, is that you can only help someone who is willing to be helped. They need to be discontent with where they are at and they need to be unafraid to look into the heart of darkness.

A person whose intent is to be ill will remain ill, even if they have not yet realized that this is their intent.

Exercise:

What is your intent for your life?
What is all of your life telling you that your secret intent for your life really is?
What is in your heart of darkness?

Chapter Seven:

The art of Healing (the what)

I know God will not give me anything I can't handle. I just wish that He didn't trust me so much. - **Mother Teresa**

Metatronic Energy works through intent. Your intention for the body and the spirit will decide what this energy does. Make your intention what you truly want it to be.

I keep my desires for a person out of a session, or my thoughts about the rightness or the wrongness of what they want or feel, or believe, and then we will get a much better result. I won't give them complex systems, or spiritual reasons, or angelic lessons. I will explain what to do and why to do it, then I will drop Metatronic Energy into them, along an agreed pathway, and let it all go. My intent is what they want. If they want to walk again, after struggling to walk, I will place that intent. If they intend to be unwell and they do not agree to change that intent, I cannot change it for them.

People are the great unknown in healing.

I have seen people who have originally come to me in a wheelchair, walk back in to see me. They have walked in using a walking stick, but they were still walking and they were happy for that result.

The results that we (Metatron and I) get with this energy are not 'miraculous' but they are human, and see-able. When I am unwell I will drop Metatronic Energy in to heal me. I will not immediately leap from my bed shouting 'Hallelujah! I am completely cured!', though that disappoints me. My body is human. It needed time to adjust to being well again. It needed time for the pathways to be rebuilt in my brain when I healed my brain damage.

The energy is instant, the healing is instant, but the results took time to implement and to show. The body needs time to catch up.

Healing and Balance

We know that the body and the spirit are separate living forces. They interact beautifully and mostly fully, but they are separate, and you have to heal both of them to achieve balance. Without balance, nothing will work.

How do we heal using Metatronic Energy?

The simplest explanation is to tell you that you talk or think about your situation and your conversation with yourself or others will create a reaction in the corresponding cells. This is like irradiating those cells so that the Metatronic Energy can find the correct cells to go to.

All the cells of the body communicate with each other as well as the cells of other beings and other life forms. It is a beautiful and complex dance of life that we are constantly involved in. The swing and the sweep of energy, intent and balance. It is fantastic to watch.

In the body, because of your discussion, there is now a pathway, a road map, a line drawn that goes into organs, muscles, bones, tissues, blood and cells. It also, this line, crosses into chakras and the auric field. Wherever there is a trace of the dysfunction that you are working on, the path has been laid.

You, the balancer, the facilitator, the healer, then calls Metatronic Energy in and it sweeps through the body and follows that path that you have laid.

You do not need to keep the energy going. You do not need to stand there and put more energy in. You have set up the resonance and the body will naturally pull in as much or as little as it needs. Just like taking a vitamin pill, the body will absorb what it needs and will excrete what is too much for it.

You cannot overdose on this energy, you cannot use too much, or too little. It just cannot happen.

What will Metatronic Energy do?

Metatronic Energy will repair and balance the body and then it will empty the toxins, or the stories, from the body and the chakras. You are then given the opportunity to replace that old, unwanted stuff with new and happier memories.

Metatronic Energy will do all this is a very short space of time. One hour is as long as I take in a session, to talk, to plan, to run the energy and then to teach you how to handle the results, because remember, you are part of this, also.

The actual Metatronic Energy will keep on working for as long as it is needed. If that is a day, it will go for a day, if that is a month, it will continue. When I healed my brain I dropped one dose of Metatronic Energy and I did not use it again for about five months. It just kept working.

Carmel Bell

The finer points of Healing

I do not like the word healer because it puts the onus on me, when it should be on you. You are the one thing that I cannot control, that nobody can control, unless you want to be controlled. I hear you winding up to argue with me about all the times that you have done things that you did not want to do, because someone 'made you'. Consider this –Viktor Frankl, the father of psychotherapy and seriously one of my heroes spent some time in a concentration camp, which is how he devised his profession. He discovered that even though he was in a concentration camp, told what to eat and what to wear. Told where he could walk, talk, sleep, and work. He, like many others, was told how he could live. He had *absolutely no freedom and no rights* but Viktor discovered that no-one could tell him what to feel. He had complete, total choice about how he responded and felt. Even if they told him when and where to dance, they could not control how he felt about it.

You see, you really are the most powerful being at the centre of the Universe, because we all know that the Universe revolves around you. You create what happens to you by choosing how you feel and how you respond. When I 'heal' you I cannot guarantee any miracle results because I cannot guarantee *you.*

The truth is no one heals anybody else. Your body heals itself, with assistance. I am a Medical Intuitive. But for the ease of simplicity, we will continue to use the word healer in this book, but also understand that healer means balancer, and facilitator and releaser. It means all of these things.

Seriously. Nobody heals anybody else. You heal yourself. Let's just look at some more facts.

You have an infection and you take antibiotics, but they do not always work. Why not?

You are tired and you pop a few Vitamin B's. Does that help? Not always.

You have torn muscles in your shoulder and the surgeon repairs it. Are you guaranteed success? Never. You are told of the percentages and there is an expected failure rate.

It is an odds game. The wild card in this fabulous game called life is YOU. See, back to you. It is up to you to accept the healing, to prepare the body, to search out the reasons why you became ill in the first place.

These are the reasons why I always talk to you when you come to see me. I am searching for the reasons why you are not well and then the reasons why you may choose to refuse to heal, and then, possibly slightly more confusing, what it is that is stopping you healing and that *you did not even know was there*! By talking to you I am doing something that you are not even aware of which is pulling to the surface all those painful moments and terrible memories and unforgivable sins that you thought you had forgotten. I am talking to you about them, pulling them out and drawing attention to them once more, so that when I put Metatronic Energy into your body, it will seek these moments out.

If you remove these moments, these memories, these toxins, then the body has room, has ability and has the desire to repair and balance back to health.

Your body has a natural need to be in balance, which is why you suffer from pain whenever you are in a state of imbalance. This is true whether it is a physical, an emotional or a spiritual imbalance.

Any time you have pain of any sort, pay attention and ask yourself 'Why?'

Look again for that space in between and find the answer.

Morality

We are going to talk about the moralities of healing. When someone comes to me for healing, they have given me permission to help them, but even so I still ask them if they want the healing. I tell them what I am going to do, as I wrote about in the first client session we discussed. I tell them what class of issues we are targeting and I ask them if that is okay.

I would have seen more than 10,000 people so far in my career and I would have taught maybe as many as 3000 people in my Funshops and of that number I can only remember one person refusing a healing at the end of the session. They said that they were not ready to let go.

This person came back for a second session and went ahead with the healing.

I never send remote healing to anyone, unasked. If another person asks me to send healing, I refuse.

I also refuse to discuss another person in session without their permission. Even children over the age of

16 and often over the age of 14 I will not discuss without their permission and then only to their parent/guardian. I will also always check with a person before I send a letter or a report to their doctor.

I have a block on my energy system so that unrequested healing goes away without bothering me, I usually won't even notice it being sent.

I consider it to be extremely rude for someone to send healing to me because they decided I need it. What if they have a different agenda to me for me? What if they think that they know better than me as to what I need or want? That is fairly common. Every profession suffers from such arrogance and the healing profession is no exception.

On occasion I have had healers say to me, "I tried to send you healing last night, but it was blocked." Or "I asked your Higher Self and it said no." They say it as a way of complaining.

I am very grateful for healing and I often will ask another healer to send me some energy. I will *ask*. Do not ask my Higher Self or anybody else's. Ask me, ask them. Give me and them the respect of knowing what they do or do not want. If you do not know them well enough to ask, you should not be sending any energy.

The exception to this may be when there has been a disaster with multiple tragedies and the general area needs some help. Many people will send energy as a collective to a collective.

My energy system has been instructed to block everything that I have not asked for, regardless of intent. After all, what is an attack, but unrequested energy?

It is bad manners to send healing to someone else without their express permission.

Healer; heal thyself and keep your intentions out of me.

Even when I was in hospital recently, one of the first people that came to see me was my friend, Enzo, who does all the psychic attack clearings for me. He placed shields around me immediately so that all unrequested healings would be sent away.

Some of my rules are:
- Do not talk about another person to somebody else. Keep your client confidentiality.
- Do not heal another person without their direct consent. If they are in a coma, or otherwise incapable of giving permission, ask their carer for permission.
- Never read another person's energy without their permission. That is the same as reading their diary.
- Never seek to control another human through fair means, or foul.

Integrity

As a healer one expects that you will have integrity.

What is integrity?

The definition in the dictionary is an 'adherence to moral and ethical principles; soundness of moral character; honesty.' Lots of people say they have integrity.

And I do not dispute them. But I do not always know what their moral and ethical standards are.

When you use this word, integrity, as a defence against something that you have done, are about to do, or say you cannot do, or cannot agree with, be sure of what you mean.

My integrity says that I do not kill another human, but a cannibal would have a different level of integrity and are they wrong? Well – no. They are not wrong. You and I may like to think that they are wrong. But we are not in their position. And sometimes we excuse murder, such as if someone was about to murder our child, we may murder them to save our child. This is a tricky situation. There is no clear answer for some things. You do not steal but what if you are starving, have no money and need to feed your family?

So, I think it is important for you to understand what integrity means to you and to live your life based on that for you, but to deal with other people on their level of integrity. If they want to come live in your home, it is reasonable to expect them to honor your code. But if you are helping them to heal, it is not reasonable for you to force your code on them.

Be clear about where you stand and what integrity means to you.

Failure

Ah, the big one. Failure. Who isn't afraid of failure? I say that if you are going to do something, do it well. Fail spectacularly!

But don't let a fear of failing drag you down. We all have failures. Some people just won't get well. This is something that you need to learn to not take personally. You simply cannot be everything to everybody and you simply cannot make everything better for all.

Hey – even God gets yelled at. Even scientists make mistakes. Everybody has to take a deep breath and shrug.

If you are not prepared to fail, you cannot succeed.

Exercise:

I would like you to consider where you have failed and what you learnt from that failure.

Chapter Eight:

Seeing Energy

It takes as much energy to wish as it does to plan.
- Eleanor Roosevelt

Everyone is intuitive. If you feel that you're not, you do perhaps not understand what intuition is. The exercises will help you to trust your intuition more, and to feel energy. It's okay. I like to have proof, which is why I start you out feeling Energy. I have never done anything just because I was told to, and I don't expect you to, either.

You may find that you're drawn to certain exercises and that you feel better after you perform them. The exercises in this book are natural and they can help you.

I hope that this book will show you that you're much more than you think you are and that your potential for growth is real. I also want to introduce you to Metatronic Energy.

Important: *this book is not meant to be used to replace your physician and medical treatment. If you're currently under the care of a doctor, follow their instructions. If you're ill, see your doctor and be guided by them.*

Carmel Bell

Seeing Energy

The very first and really handy skill to develop is how to see energy. You will probably be amazed at how easy it is to see. You may even realize that you have already been seeing it for years. You just may need to recognize it, or refine it.

Some people will see energy with their eyes, as I do. Other people will see energy in their mind, as an overlay on a person or thing. That is okay as well. Some people hear or feel energy and I have met people who smell it or taste it. Whatever does it for you.

A case study

About 15 years ago I was training a gentleman, Joseph, to see and feel energy. Joseph wanted to be an energy healer, or spiritual healer, and as with everything, I believe that it is better to 'know' than to be told. So with this in mind, I told him that I would teach him to see energy before I did anything else.

For weeks, Joseph sat in class with me and my other students. He would stare, unblinking for as long as he could at the other students, until his eyes watered and I was not sure if he was crying or not. Joseph understood why I wanted him to see the energy for himself, but he felt such despair and hopelessness at ever being able to. It got to the point where I told him to just relax and that if it did not happen this week, we would move on without it.

Joseph was despondent that night when he left to go home. I wondered if I would ever see him again. The very next day the phone rang and when I answered it, it was a very excited Joseph on the other end.

"I can see!" He exclaimed loudly, "I can see!" It seems that he was at his work, in the cafeteria having lunch. Joseph was really not trying, he was tired and he was hungry, so he was just sitting quietly eating and staring at space. In front of him was one of his co-workers, also sitting and eating quietly. Neither was paying attention to the other person. This lack of attention did the trick. Out of the corners of his eyes, Joseph could suddenly see a heat haze kind of light wafting and pulsing around his co-workers' head. It was very bright and see-through, yet kind of grey. This heat haze/light kept disappearing and then coming back, like it was pulsating. The more Joseph took notice of it, the more it disappeared, yet when he ignored it, it came back.

Joseph had done it! He had given up trying, relaxed and as a result, he had seen what he was trying to see. Energy is delicate and shy. Just when you think energy will never appear, it does. Once you have learnt to recognize it, it becomes less shy and you will realize that you have been seeing it all your life.

Carmel Bell

What does seeing Energy look like?

You *can* learn to see energy. It is like seeing a mirage on the road when you are driving. And it usually only requires a little bit of training to make it show to you.

Understand that repressing your intuitive skills is a mistake. Your intuition is a completely natural sense, just like your sight and hearing and if you repress it it's as if you're wearing blinkers. Intuition is a sense as much as sight, hearing and touch are senses. It's meant to help you.

Our society is set up to make it difficult for you. Energy is a light source, but a very subtle and diffused light source. Like a candle flame, the more brightly lit the environment that light is in, the less able to see it you will be. It is amazing how many people struggle emotionally when they are in an artificially lit environment. Look at the SAD syndrome: people who suffer from depression during winter when most of the lighting around them is artificial. These people need sunlight to feel happy. They need summer time, and sunshine, or sunlamps to bring a smile to their face.

And how many people feel better when they are in a candle lit environment? Think about the lighting around you and don't always cover yourself in glare.

Energy is very easy to see in sunlight and it can be quite hard to see under fluorescent lighting.

Seeing Energy around plants and trees.

Let me start with the fundamentals of what energy is and what it is not.

With each energetic exercise, I teach you I want you to use your intention to ask for what you want to achieve.

Thoughts create reality. I think therefore I am.

When viewing energy, ask to see energy. You will find what you seek, so just for a moment, quietly sit and 'intend' to see energy. Don't force it – just be patient.

This intention process will become automatic, but only after you have practiced INTENTION for a short space of time.

The first energy we are going to view is the bio-energy. This is the energy layer closest to the body. There are seven layers of energy around our bodies and the closer they are to us, the heavier, and the more physical they become. Each layer has its own purpose. This layer is your life force layer and it tells me when you are well, unwell, happy, sad, lying, telling the truth and more. Because it is so dense and so physical, it is the easiest to see.

Bio-energy is a living energy. Bio-energy pulses, in and out, in waves. It will appear to grow larger and smaller as it pulses. It will not stay the same, so just when you think you can see it, it will disappear. Relax. It will reappear. It also pulses faster or slower depending on what you are thinking about.

Prana, Chi, Orgone Energy, life force...

This is all the same energy, just named differently in different cultures. You have probably seen this energy all your life without recognizing it.

Bio-energy is often most easily seen and recognized as the little sparkles that you see floating in the air on a summer's day, or arising off trees and plants, in a haze. When this energy is in the air, we call this orgone energy and the bright sparkly bits are live orgone energy, whilst the black dots and squiggles are dead orgone energy.

Exercise One: seeing Energy around plants and trees.

First, let us go outside, if possible. It is best to have a sunny day, or at least not overcast and raining when you are starting out. Just like us, energy is more active when the sun is shining.

- Set your *intention* to see this energy.
- Put fear and expectations aside.
- Relax. Allow your eyes and your body to relax.
- Look into the air without looking at anything in particular.
- Look around the trees and past the trees, without looking *at* the tree.

- You may become aware of sparkles of energy, either silvery or dark. This energy will be sighted in your peripheral vision in the space *between* you and the tree. You may also see energy streams coming off plants. This energy stream will look like a vapor trail.
- Plants consume the 'spent' energy from us and return it renewed so that we can use it again. Just like carbon dioxide.
- Remember that this energy is 'see through', so it will be like seeing through the heat haze you will spot coming off a hot road, or the heat haze arising off a gas flame.
- Remember that as soon as you focus on the particles of energy, they will fade.

Seeing Human Energy

The human energy system is made up of both the energetic body and the physical body.

The two bodies, energetic and physical, interact on an inseparable level and what happens in one is then reflected in the other. They create each other and are created by each other. Of course, you already see your physical body, so let us now turn your attention to seeing the energetic body.

For those readers who may be vision impaired, you can do the same thing, view energy, with your third eye vision, if you have a memory of how the body looked. Or if you have been vision impaired all your life, or you have no particular sight memory, you can also feel/see with your hands. The human energy system may feel smooth and in other parts, sticky or prickly. It may feel hot, cold, invigorating, nauseating, and many other feelings. I will sometimes use my hands if someone is so low in energy that it is very hard to see them.

To help you learn, I will talk about the basics of the human energy system for you.

The Human Energy System

The Physical

People commonly believe that the body is a solid object but in reality the physical body is a collection of molecules that have clustered together enough to be seen by the eye. Their density creates the appearance of the physical body. These molecules are made up from the same energy as everything else in the Universe, including thoughts and emotions.

In fact, scientists in Copenhagen, led by Professor Eugene Polzik and using Quantum mechanics, magnetism and a process that they call Quantum Entanglement, have managed to move energy 'information'.

Quantum entanglement relies on the fact that two photons can be created in such a way that they behave as a single object, even if they are separated by large distances. In behaving this way they act as a teleportation machine because any change to one causes similar changes in the other. The way that this is done is via a third photon, which is teleported from the photon in the transmitting station to the photon in the receiver. However, this does mean that whatever is transported is actually a copy and not the original item or information.

The third photon carries the information with it to the receiving photon, via Quantum information. The third photon then becomes identical to the first photon. Hence, the information is transported successfully.

Albert Einstein described Quantum Entanglement as "spooky action at a distance".

(I'll just interject here, without Albert Einstein, we energy healers would be quite lost. We have been given more interesting and fascinating quotes than almost anyone. Well done, Albert! My thanks.)

Research also continues at the University of Vienna, led by Professor Robert Ursin.

In essence – our bodies are not solid, unchanging objects. Our thoughts create our reality and our emotions create our body.

At times what we see can hurt us, what we cannot see can help us.

The common belief is that what we can see we can deal with and that "what we don't know can't hurt us." As a result we usually do not deal with the unseen energy, waiting instead until we become ill before dealing with the results. Energy medicine is designed to help you deal with the results before you suffer the effects. If you become aware of your emotions, your thoughts and your body – so dealing with the physical and the spiritual – you can prevent or lessen the impact on the physical.

The Spiritual

Expanding out from the physical body is another less dense collection of molecules that we call the aura or the human energy system.

Einstein taught us that matter and energy are essentially interchangeable and their transformations are eternally continuous. All matter is energy. The chair you are sitting in, the clothes you are wearing and the thoughts you are thinking are made of energy. This energy is indestructible.

Einstein's work also taught us that no matter how small energy particles are; they are as eternal as the vastness of the Universe. There is no lower limit to the quantity of action that is needed to effect any change. In other words, a minute amount of energy may be just as effective in bringing about a change as is a large amount of energy.

The aura also has systems that mimic and are mimicked by the physical body. These energetic systems transport the spiritual, emotional and energetic information as well as the physical information throughout our bodies, on all levels.

These energetic systems within the aura also transport the unseen component of *every moment and experience in our life.* Imagine how important and powerful this really is. It is this subtle energy that is the unseen cause behind every illness we experience and also every moment of wellness. It is here, if we know how, that we can first locate, diagnose, prevent and heal dysfunction

– regardless of whether that is mental, physical or spiritual in origin.

Energy medicine is a core component to our health and well being. It is impossible to be free of the energy body, even after death because when you are dead, all you are is energy! The energy body creates your physical body and also dictates the types of experiences you attract. Your physical body and the experiences you have undergone also create the energy body. It is a two-way street.

The Aura – The Physical

What it is...

The auric field is a pulsing, electromagnetic field that completely surrounds, penetrates, and covers the body.

The auric field comprises of seven layers that reflect the physical body and your health. These layers both emanate from, and create the electromagnetic energy that your body discharges.

The aura is a living, breathing part of your body that will change as quickly as you do and will reflect your health, your thoughts, and your fears. Your aura is completely unique to you. It holds the 'blueprint' of all your life and it is not unusual to find damage in the aura years after it has been healed in the physical body. It is this damage being held in the auric field that creates weakness and dysfunction in the body, allowing further illness. Once an illness has moved beyond potential, into actual and is impacting the body, both the auric field and the body need to be repaired. We need to deal with every illness holistically. As Caroline Myss so beautifully phrased for us, "Your Biography becomes your Biology."

- Every living being has an aura.
- The aura is an electromagnetic field ranging from infrared to ultraviolet.
- Every living cell has an aura – be that from a human, animal, plant, or mineral.
- The aura moves in and through and around the body.

How the Bio Energy/Aura behaves...

- It will move in and out, like a wave.
- It will flow closer to and further away from, the body (think pulsing).
- It is affected by emotion and thought.
- It will pulse like an electromagnetic flow.
- It is affected by disease.
- It flows from the right to the left.

What the Aura is not...

- It is not static.
- It is not caused by imagination.
- It is not a mirage.
- And will not stay the same – ever.

- It is not invulnerable.

What colour is the Aura?

The aura is no particular color. It is seen as a colour because colours are an energy frequency and we see the aura as the same sort of energy frequency.

Think of a spectrum of light, infra red rays or ultra violet light. Our eyes see these signals as a colour wave.

The colours in your aura change all the time as they are reflecting different thoughts, feelings, emotions, and issues. Your aura is no colour and all colours.

What do we use the Aura for?

We use the aura to find and correct dysfunction and ailments. The aura will hold and show where in the body there is disease. The chakras hold the reason you got sick.

Exercise Two: seeing Human Energy

Seeing energy – bio-energy around a human.

There are three ways to see energy– which one is for you?

1. Seeing the bio-energy physically with your eyes.

2. Seeing the bio-energy intuitively with your third eye.
3. Knowing/sensing the bio-energy.

The bio-energy is easy to see. The chances are that you have been seeing and ignoring this energy for all of your life. Some people are more comfortable seeing this energy in their mind. Bio-energy is basically the same as what we call a mirage or heat haze on a road. If you can see this, you can learn to see the bio-energy

Seeing the bio-energy is a little more challenging than seeing the energy around plants and trees, largely because of feelings of fear and a fragile self esteem. The method of viewing is the same. Many people will see only brief glimpses of the bio-energy, many more will only see the bio-energy in their third eye space.

Be gentle with yourself. It is fantastic to use every tool available to see energy.

A few suggestions:

You need a partner for this exercise, or if you cannot find someone to practice with, try lying down and holding your hand up in front of your face, at arm's length, so that you can see your hand against the ceiling – most ceilings are plain coloured.

You can also be out in a public place and just casually look at someone. You may see the aura.

Or even at the movie theatre, sometimes the aura shows up really well when you can see the top of the head of the person in the row in front of you. The light from the screen, your relaxed state and their relaxed state, will sometimes show it up quite nicely.

For the background

- Use subdued lighting. Your lights should be turned down a bit, but brighter than candle light.
- A clean, non-patterned backdrop is best if you can choose. A solid colour, sometimes lighter is better when you are starting out.
- Try to have about 30 cm between your partner and the wall to allow you to have some empty space between the wall and the bio-energy.
- Position yourself at a distance from your partner. Two metres or more is ideal.

For technique

- Relax. You can do it!
- Ignore the energy – the harder you search for it, the more it will sometimes resist your attempts.
- Look at the head and shoulder area, as this is where the energy will most likely be the strongest.
- Sometimes it helps to observe from the side of your eyes, otherwise known as peripheral vision.

What you should start to see

You should start to notice a heat haze or a 'reverse shadow' effect.

Look around close to the body. You will notice that the immediate area around the head and shoulders is brighter than the area beyond it. In other words, the area in between the shadow and the body will be brighter. It will probably be a very thin line of brightness.

You should then start to see pale, 'washed out' energy. It will probably look similar to water colour paint that has been washed lightly over glass – the colour or energy is not solid and is see through.

This energy will usually disappear almost as soon as it appears. Remember that all energy pulses in and out.

Do not expect energy to sit stagnant and wait for you to notice it. Talk, interact, play. The energy will shift, flow, increase, and decrease as you speak.

Watch the energy appear and disappear. Watch how some topics increase the energy and other topics will diminish it.

Why are we viewing the Bio-Energy of the Aura?

Because this is the layer that will tell us how vital, how alive we are.

This is very important. Even if you cannot see any other energy layer on yourself or the person you are viewing with your physical eyes, you can still discern how well, how happy and how invested a person is through this layer. You can also tell by the changes in the bio-energy which are the more important emotional issues to a person.

If you cannot see this energy, you can still feel it. Use your hands but don't touch the body. Feel where over the body the energy may feel smooth, or slippery, or sticky, or prickly. There are lots of ways that it may feel.

Beyond the bio-energy there are other layers in the aura.

Emotional layer: multi-coloured.

Mental layer: varies from yellow to orange.

Astral or causal layer: multi-coloured also. This is the layer that holds all the information about your physical and emotional ailments. It is the connector between the physical and the spiritual.

Etheric Blueprint: This is the layer in which you can actually restructure the body and effect really good repairs.

Celestial: this layer is the Universal connection

Ketheric: the Divine layer. This connects you to spirit.

Chapter Nine:

Feeling Energy

It takes a lot more energy to fail than to succeed, since it takes a lot of concentrated energy to hold on to beliefs that don't work. - **Jerry Gillies**

Everything is energy, even rocks and stones, which seem completely inanimate to us. I am going to teach you to feel energy. Remember, energy is subtle. It is not going to feel like a marauding pack of spiders stomping across your hand, or blocks of ice that you might hold. It will feel light and gentle. Some people feel it as a tickle, other people feel it as a cold breeze, yet others will feel it as warm energy. However you feel or experience it is okay. There is no right way or wrong way to feel energy.

The human energy system has been known about and acknowledged for thousands of years. In India, life energy is called prana and healing by working with the energy system is known as Pranic Healing. In China, life energy is called chi, and healing using the energy system is called Chi Kung or Qi Gong healing. And out of Japan we were given the magnificent energy called Reiki.

India's Pranic Healing is known to many practitioners of yoga who practice pranayama exercises and Chi Kung has become popular worldwide as a method of regaining health by working with chi energy. Even in western societies, we use PET scans, CAT scans, Kirlian photography and thermal imaging to measure energy. This energy is what we are going to start off feeling.

Try this simple exercise. We are going to feel this energy through your hands. Why your hands? Your hands contain the most sensitive energy points of your body and you are used to feeling through your hands.

Exercise Three: Feeling Energy

- Choose a time and a place where you can have some quiet and some calmness. It is probably not a good idea to do this at work, or just before dinner on a school night. And you won't have to do this every time, but it will help you to have a quiet place whilst you are learning to recognize energy.
- I want you to relax. Sit or stand comfortably and shake your shoulders loose. Now shake your arms and let the gentle vibration travel down your arms into your hands.
- Relax your hands. Open them, close them, open them again. Give them a brisk shake to make sure the blood if flowing. Just for a second, but not so hard that all you can feel is tingles! If you go that far, relax again and wait for the tingles to stop.

And finally, we are here. The moment has arrived! I want you to set your intent to feel energy.

- Gently, but rapidly, rub your hands together for about 30 seconds. You are not trying to start a fire, just open your palm chakras.
- Give your hands a gentle clap together.
- Now move your hands a few inches apart and then move them closer together again, slowly, so they are close – but not touching. The fingertips may touch, or they may not. You should feel a slight resistance in between your palms, like you might expect to feel if you were holding a thin, lightly inflated balloon.
- Move your hands closer together and then further apart again a few times. See how well you can feel that gentle push between your hands. A springy, slightly full energy that is pushing your hands away from each other.
- You'll be able to feel the energy around and between your hands. It's palpable. This is your own life energy.
- If you feel like it, pop the energy that you are now playing with into the top of your head, or onto a plant. Don't waste it.

This energy is as real as you are. This energy is around everybody and every part of your body. It helps to form your own warning system of when someone has come to close to you for comfort, for instance. We all react and innately read this energy as it comes off each other.

I often just ask for energy and I will feel it on the top of my head where it will then flow down through my crown chakra and into my body. I will know it is working because I will also usually get a gentle shiver through my body.

As you become more familiar with your life energy, you can use it to enhance your health. For example, if you suffer from indigestion, or other stomach troubles, just pull some energy onto your hands, and then place your hands against your stomach. This is a very simple form of self healing. It will not repair your body but it will help to relieve pain.

In Chi Kung, students are told that chi, life energy, follows attention. You may already know this: that whatever you place your attention on grows. If you focus on the negative, you'll get more of what you don't want. Focus on the positive and the positive elements of your life will grow too.

All illness and disease affects your energy system before it affects your physical body. An intuitive healer can see your energy system. Sometimes they can read what illnesses are affecting you now and which illnesses may affect you soon because they're already in your energy system.

As you work with the exercises in this book, you'll get to know your energy system, and how to work with it.

Chapter Ten:

Grounding and Sealing

Energy can be wild, untamed and erratic if it is not kept in check. Very few people are grounded into the earth.

You have learnt to see, and to feel and to call bio-energy. Now I invite you to learn how to maintain yourself before we try Metatronic Energy.

The human body is made up of Electromagnetic Energy, or a form of electricity, which is why you sometimes get a little shock of things when you touch them, or walking on nylon carpet can cause a shock. Have you ever thought about sleeping on a mattress with inner springs under you and the effect that this would be having on your body? I, personally, sleep on latex...

We all are reasonably familiar with the idea that electricity needs to be grounded to be safe. Aren't we?

So – here we live inside a big electromagnetic energy body, discharging electricity all the time. Let's ground it.

Grounding from the body to the Universe and to the Earth so that you are connected to all happens through the base chakra.

The base chakra sits on the perineum, which is the area of flesh in between your genitals and your anus.

The base chakra is red in its 'energy signal'. This is not because it is actually red, sometimes it is all different sorts of colours, when it goes off balance. But that is its signature. 1000-2000hz Red.

Why do we ground?

When we talk about grounding, we are talking about recalling your energy from the past and back from the future, into the HERE and NOW inside your body. The more you are concerned with how you were in the past, or how things may progress in the future, the less likely you are to be healthy. Your body needs you to be as PRESENT as possible. Grounding, via the following method will make you as strong as possible energetically.

The base chakra is designed to ground you to keep you energetically inside yourself, away from the past and from worry about the future, so that you are here, and you can concentrate on the NOW.

Exercise Four: Grounding

- In your mind SEE, FEEL or IMAGINE a small red circle about four inches in diameter. Just see this red circle in the space where you might imagine an image of something you like, for instance. This red circle will AUTOMATICALLY locate to the base chakra because they are of the same frequency so there is NO NEED for you to see it on the base chakra.
- Now out of the underneath of this circle allow a cord of ANY COLOUR to grow down about three

feet in length. You will end up with something that may look like a balloon with a string hanging down, or a flower with a stem. Or a flat disc with a cord.
- Then see/feel or imagine a small patch of EARTH or even a patch of grey, or somewhere that you like, such as your garden at home. DO NOT try to Ground into the earth where you sit because it is hard to ground 20,000 feet if you are on a plane, for instance. Keep the whole grounding procedure in your mind.
- Allow the cord to touch the earth. The cord will automatically start to grow roots. Then let the image go, knowing that you will stay grounded.
- You may need to ground several times a day. Sometimes you may need to ground several times in a row.
- Whenever you are feeling anxious, tired, off balance or are having trouble sleeping – try grounding. If you cannot 'see' the above procedure, saying it in your mind will work just as well. Your *intention* will set the GROUNDING. All you need say is "Small red circle, Cord, patch of Earth."

Well done. You are grounded. The next thing that you want to do is to keep yourself sealed. I have heard many excuses for people not wanting to seal themselves. I have seen many a person get ill out of being unsealed.

Sealing is as much about you keeping others safe as it is about you keeping you safe.

Exercise Five: Sealing

When I talk about sealing I am talking about an energy level that will keep you safe from other HUMAN energy systems. Sealing is important whilst you are going through a healing and release process because it will help stop you from 'throwing' your issues at others and also from reacting to other people responses to your altered system.

Over my career I have had many people argue with me about the need to seal. Most of those people, to be fair, were idealistic and altruistic. They did not really have a clue. You are not sealing so that you will not feel. You are not sealing because everything is radically unsafe. You are sealing to set boundaries between you and everybody else.

Sealing gives you the ability to choose. Choose how you feel, how you react, where you place your attention and your energy.

Have you ever walked into a shopping centre, only to get exhausted or gone to a party, only to find yourself off balance? Do you pick up other people's feelings far too easily, so easily in fact, that you cannot decide sometimes how you feel?

Or walked in feeling fine and left soon after with a headache, or feeling unwell?

All of these examples are indicative of the need to seal your energy system. When I meet you, I want to meet you, not a version of me, or the person standing next to me. You.

- We SEAL with the vibration of GOLD.
- This is best and most quickly done by imagining a bucket of GOLD liquid pouring over our head. Keep this gold seal as close as possible to your body. Many people use a bubble but if you use a bubble, each time someone comes close to you they are within your SEAL. Think about a shopping centre, or a train trip…

Chapter Eleven:

Metatronic Energy - an experiment

'You tell someone you're a Metatron, they stare at you blankly. You mention something out of a Charlton Heston movie and suddenly everyone is a theology scholar!'
- from '**Dogma**'

You have felt energy and hopefully played with it for a while, rolling the ball around. You have learned to ground and seal yourself and we have talked about all sorts of issues, some of which may have made you happy, while other issues may have made you uncomfortable. The cunning plan behind all this, is this has been laying little energy pathways through your body, bouncing from one chakra point to another. Hmmm, there are only seven chakras, right? No. There are 365 of them, all over your body. Think about acupuncture points. They tend to mimic chakras.

I want to introduce you to Metatronic Energy. I want you to be aware of this energy and how it works, so that you can choose to learn about it. I tossed and turned about whether or not I should try to teach you via a book to feel this amazing energy and the thing is, if you have never felt any energy at all, what you *do* manage to feel will probably feel pretty amazing, which means essentially, you will be able to mistake that energy for Metatronic Energy, but I will not be able to be *certain* that you have felt Metatronic Energy. I like to teach people myself and it is very easy to find once you have been attuned to it – but I have never attuned people to it through a book before.

Even so, I think that we will try with the idea of you learning Metatronic Energy through this book. I will tell you what it feels like and how to ask for it, but if you want to be certain that you have found Metatronic Energy; you need to be given Metatronic Energy in person. Please contact me through my website at www.carmelbell.com.au and we, my assistants and I, will see if we can organise a Funshop for you in your area.

A Breakdown

Metatronic Energy is an angelic energy. When I say 'an angelic energy', I encourage you to not see some person floating about with wings and a harp and then tell yourself how beautiful it all is. Angels are as real as us; they are different to us. Their needs, wants, desires and life times go into something different to us. In my experience from being in Heaven with angels, I noticed that they are more powerful than us and their energy is more capable of altering a structure or dysfunction in your body. They stand between you and God/That Which Is and they transmute that energy so that you can feel it, without being destroyed.

By comparison, all bio-energy, which is so well known around the world, for very good reason, is a human energy. This does not mean that it is not as good as Metatronic Energy, it does mean though, that it is used for different things and in my experience, I have found it to be slower working. Sometimes you need to go slow.

And when I say human, I do not mean that it comes out of a human body. I mean that it will pass through a human body, it is easier to find for humans and angels are not likely to be using it. Though some of the more basic bio-energy does come out of a human body, which is the same energy that trees and plants use to heal and to grow.

These sorts of energies are equal to each other but they are different to each other. It is like saying that red and purple are both colours, but we understand they are not the *same* colour. When we measure them on instruments that are designed for that purpose, we find that these colours have different frequencies to each other. Infrared and ultraviolet, for instance are the two ends of the known spectrum from each other.

Energies that align closely to the base, sacral, and solar plexus chakra energies are more 'human' and energies that align closer to the throat, third eye and crown are angelic in frequency. All energy passes through the heart chakra.

When I am tired, depressed, or can't sleep, for instance, I use a bio-energy on myself. But when I want to know *why* I am tired, depressed or can't sleep, I use Metatronic Energy.

This is another really significant key point to the difference between these energies. Metatronic Energy is a curious and what can only be best described as an intelligent energy.

An intelligent energy? You have never thought of energy as something that has a consciousness? Of course energy does. Everything does. Every cell in your body has a consciousness. That does not mean that each cell has a separate identity, but it knows when it is sick. Research scientists know that cells will deliberately choose to let themselves die when they are sick. That this is, in fact, their actual function – to choose to die when sick. Everything has a consciousness. So does energy. And even more so, so does Metatronic Energy. It wants to work in concert with you, for the best result from a healing. This is why the way that I work and train includes energy involvement.

What is Metatronic Energy?

Metatronic Energy is a healing energy and a repairing energy. You may already be aware of Reiki, Pranic, or other healing energies. These fabulous energies are *similar* but very *different* from Metatronic Energy, much like a rally car is similar but very different to a Formula One race car.

Metatronic Energy will not stop you from dying and nor is it meant to. Dying is part of life and it is a wonderful part of life, but Metatronic Energy will help you to live the best life possible for you, accepting responsibility for every moment of your life. Essentially, it will help you to be the author of your own existence.

Metatronic Energy is a different frequency to anything else you have experienced so far. It is designed to be used for a different purpose. Most other frequencies will give you the energy you need to live your life. Metatronic Energy is designed to rebuild and repair your energy system so that you *can* live. This is why it was able to repair my brain, something that is currently outside of medical and scientific paradigms. It is not that it is untestable and unexplainable. Metatronic Energy is actually very testable and explainable. It is just that it has not yet been very tested. But it will be.

I use Metatronic Energy when I am unwell, on any level. I use what I call bio-energy when I am tired and I need some more life force.

In Heaven I was told that Metatronic Energy is needed on Earth at this present time. Metatronic Energy is intelligent, healing and restoring. It can help anyone who asks to receive it. It helps both the body, as it did with me and it helps the mind and as we are having a world epidemic of depression and anxiety, Metatronic Energy could not have come for you to use at a better time. The really exciting thing about Metatronic Energy is that it does not require secret symbols or wonderful hand movements to use it. I am an Asperger and I do not like anything that looks kind of weird. I like things to be neat, quick and repeatable, with the minimum of fuss. Metatronic Energy is perfect for me.

My intent is to explain what Metatronic Energy feels like to me and therefore how it might feel to you, as well. And then I will explain how you might find it for your own use. But I cannot guarantee that you will find it through this book. Even if you find an energy and you think that it may be Metatronic Energy, I cannot be sure that it is. This is why I prefer to teach people in person how to feel for it. This is the only way that I can be sure, for both you and me, that you have found Metatronic Energy.

We will talk about the morality of not interfering with someone else's life by sending unrequested healing later on.

My intent is also *not* to teach you to be a Medical Intuitive. To become a Medical Intuitive you need training and people to support you. I hope that some of the clients I have spoken about have shown you that this can be an interesting job, but it is not an easy job. It is a rewarding job, yes, but people are relying on you. Some will have life-threatening conditions; others will have life destroying conditions. You will win, you will lose. You will grieve, you will celebrate. Yes, I know that I had no training, but that made it harder for me, not easier. I had no one to train me, not because I am 'so special' but because there was no one there to do the training, so spirit asked me to train others. That was my original contract. I fulfilled it when I taught many people and when I set up the College of Medical Intuition that people could enrol in and come to, to learn.

Medical Intuitives have as much responsibility as doctors do, to maintain a sense of honour, integrity and truth. I have trained myself in anatomy and physiology, drugs and drug interactions, herbs, vitamins, multiple diseases, surgical procedures, psychological conditions and much more. I can only understand what is in my mind to understand. That is the purpose behind training. Then I use my intuition to tell me where to look, what has created the condition and what will improve the condition. In short, I became a Medical Intuitive.

So – my purpose is *not to train* you as a Medical Intuitive through this book. But if you feel that you have a calling to be one, contact me at my college.

I hope you'll use the exercises in this book. I know that when you do, they will improve your life in all areas.

What does Metatronic Energy feel like?

It feels like a light, sparkling energy. It feels cool and sparkling and smooth. It can feel like champagne would feel like on your palm.

Remember the feeling you had when you were playing with the bio-energy? That felt like (to me) a warm, springy or spongy, solid sort of energy.

Metatronic Energy is lighter, cooler, tinglier. So if you feel the same thing as before, keep looking.

Metatronic Energy comes from, and through the Archangel Metatron. It is the highest level of energy that we can use in this world today, which I have found, anyway. This is what I used to repair my brain and if I had not used Metatronic Energy, I would still be severely brain damaged.

I am so lucky that I had access to Metatronic Energy and that I had the sense to use it and that I also did not have enough common sense, or ordinary belief, to block it when I did use it.

In terms of chakras, it is crown chakra energy, which is why it is so 'intelligent'. But that also means that it connects to the Divine.

Metatron is the angel who is closest to God. He is the voice of God and those people who talk to God are usually talking to Metatron. We are not able to talk directly to God, or That Which Is, but S/He hears every word we say and answers every prayer. Sometimes the answer is 'No'.

In my practice, I guide my patients and students to work with this energy and I'd like to help you to discover it too. This is an experiment. I've never introduced anyone to the energy through the medium of a book before. But I feel that all you have to do to receive it is to ask for it.

I am going to ask you to hold out your right hand and ask Metatron to send his energy to you. Within a few moments, you should feel a slight tickling on your palm. You may even feel something like a shiver go down through your body. Don't expect fireworks! Just sit quietly. This energy is subtle. If you're busy at work, you'll be very distracted, so choose a time when you're relaxed and in a quiet area. If you do a course with me, I will call Metatronic Energy down and place it directly onto you. That way you learn very quickly how to recognize it.

Once you feel the energy from Metatron, you can drop Metatronic Energy onto the top of your head and let it go down through your crown chakra, if you wish to. It will do what you need it to, but you can help by quietly telling yourself, in your mind, what you would like to achieve, in terms of healing.

Remember, this energy is intelligent and although it knows what you need, it also works best when you work together with knowledge. No demanding, no pleading, just a gentle request of the energy.

If you feel like it, please let me know the results you have with this experimental way of introducing you to Metatronic Energy. Send me an email to carmel@carmelbell.com.au

Exercise Six: Feeling Metatronic Energy

The first thing I want you to do is to allow any energy that you call in to land on your right hand. We do it this way because the right hand pushes away and the left hand draws in, so energy is moving around you all the time in an anti-clockwise direction.

- Find a quiet place where you can sit comfortably.
- Hold out your right hand.
- Ask to connect to Metatronic Energy.
- Visualize sparkling energy, like champagne bubbles.
- After a few moments you should feel a gentle presence on your hand.
- When you do, drop this presence onto the top of your head with your hand, and
- Relax. It will do what it needs to do. Just feel the Metatronic Energy for now.

What will Metatronic Energy do?

It will remove the story from your chakras. Metatronic Energy will remove that toxic, creating story from you so that you will be well because you will have a choice to choose how you feel. Everything you have learnt so far will be used to facilitate this.

Chapter Twelve:

The Patterns

And what is a man without energy? Nothing - nothing at all.
- Mark Twain

The chakras are the first pattern.

What are the chakras?

Chakras are energy vortices into the body. There are SEVEN major chakras that deal with all of human development and growth, and all of spiritual development and growth.

These seven major chakras vibrate to a different colour frequency each. Each one is linked to a series of smaller chakras that sit on pathways through the body. When those pathways are physical we call them meridians and when they are spiritual we call them nadis, but same thing, basically.

The chakras are where illnesses are created. They are displayed in the aura and created and stored in the chakra.

When an issue sits in a chakra, that chakra will also have lots of conditions and illnesses attached to it. If you deal with one illness, without dealing with the actual cause which is lodged in the chakra, then you will just get back the same illness, or another illness that is ruled by the same chakra. Energy must go somewhere because every moment is stored in the physical warehouse that is your body. First, the energy information about your life goes into whatever chakra is the most suitable, but when that chakra gets full, the energy still needs to be stored somewhere. It then goes into the body to be recorded as a secondary system. Because the body is not actually suited to the purpose of storage, it becomes harmed by that act, thus you develop an illness. A clever system when you think about it. The statement, your biography becomes your biology now takes on a new and invigorating truth.

When I become sick one of the first things I do is to clean out my chakras so that the information that has made me become ill has some place to be stored *other* than my body. With that taken care of, it is gratifying to see how many illnesses will revert.

Even with knowing all this, though, many people are unwilling to let go of their stories because they are concerned that they will no longer receive the secondary gain.

What does each Chakra do?

We have looked at the energy system, we have felt bio-energy and Metatronic Energy, so you should know the difference between the two energy forms. We have grounded and we have sealed.

Now you need to know what you are doing with this energy and what you can expect as a result of your work.

Following, I discuss each of the seven major chakras. The chakras are the most important part of your energy system for you to gain an understanding of, whether you work with Metatronic Energy or not. Metatronic Energy will still work, even if you do not know the pathways, but it will work better and faster when you do.

Each chakra has a different energy function, physical function and spiritual function. Every organ and every part of the body is ruled by a different chakra. Each chakra is easy to see and identify because they are different colours on the spectrum when you view them energetically and the pathway that they belong to and follow is also a different colour. It is a very quick, simple, effective and complex system.

My advice is to read about each chakra and try to remember what endocrine gland belongs to what chakra, what issues belong to what chakra and what 'power' also belongs because each chakra gains strength and sustenance from a power source. Power sources are things like energy from the Earth, energy from emotional issues, or energy from interacting with friends.

You also need to empty, or heal the chakra involved, so that it can keep storing more events without you becoming ill as the excess energy will get stored elsewhere in the body. It is a very complex and yet simple, system.

For example, and here is the interesting part - if you do not empty the chakra of the events and experiences you have undergone, you might work hard and go through therapy, recovering from alcoholism only to discover that you are now suffering from obsessive compulsive disorder instead. Of course you may blame developing OCD on no longer having the pacifier of alcohol to calm you down, but the real reason is that you are just chasing energy around inside your chakras and body until you empty the chakra of the emotional issues. In this case, as it is base it would be something connected to the family. Family can also mean work connections and friendships.

This means that every family barbecue you attended, or dinner, every time your family forgot your birthday, or you were overlooked for promotion at work, this event is stored as energy in your base chakra, primarily. This storage is invisible until it becomes physical illness, then it will become very visible.

You can actually circumvent this by recognizing the symptoms and clearing the chakra, and then, if you are truly willing to let it go, you will stand a real chance of not becoming ill.

So, worry less about what this one illness may mean and more about the pathology of the whole chakra.

Look at them as patterns and then find out what pattern you are playing, or patterns. For example, everyone who has sore bones, constipation or hemorrhoids has the base chakra pattern playing in them.

Sometimes you will have an issue that you can clearly see in your body and it will make sense. You may have been robbed and now you fear robbery – logical. But what if you have never been robbed and yet you fear robbery?

Pattern 2: Epigenetics

There is another important energy pattern you may need to consider, which is the field of Epigenetics. Epigenetics is where we carry forward into our psyche and our body, events, food preferences and even cellular changes because of things that have happened to our ancestors. Good, strong scientific research has been done into this field in recent times.

What this means, to you and I, is that sometimes you will inherit problems, preferences and a life path because of how your mother, father or grandparents were. It is worth remembering this, if you are looking at your life and things do not quite add up, such as why you believe something when you really do not want to.

Carmel Bell

The Base Chakra – Tribal Power and the power of responsibility.

Basic wants (food, water, survival)

Issues of your family – Tribal Power – family can also be work colleagues.
It is the human level of tribal/family self-identity.
Who are you seen to be, when in your family cluster? How do you fit in to your family, if you do.

Physiology of the Base Chakra

Endocrine Gland: Adrenals (flight/fight)

Body Sections ruled by the Base Chakra

Body support (skeleton, muscles, ligaments)
Spinal Column
Legs and feet
Bones
Rectum
Immune system

Mental/Emotional issues ruled by the Base Chakra

> Group safety –   being okay when you are part of a group
> Security
> Law and order
> Family issues and beliefs
> Self sufficiency
> Emotional comfortableness

Physical issues ruled by the Base Chakra

> Bed-wetting
> Candida Albicans (thrush)
> Constipation
> Depression
> Immune related disorders
> Chronic lower back pain
> Varicose veins
> Rectal cancer
> Multiple personality Disorder
> Destructive patterns
> Obsessive Compulsive Disorder
> Chronic fatigue

Purpose of the Base Chakra

Your family honor code (family can include work mates, or social club friends)
> Justice code
> Loyalty
> Group experience
> Connection to the physical world

Fears held in the Base Chakra

> Kleptomania
> Alcoholism
> Abandonment by the group
> Acting in TOXIC ways that go against your 'group'.

Energy breakdown

All of the disorders held in the base chakra have something in common - they all have fear, anger and depression as their driver and creator; fear, anger and depression that is connected to your family and other strong family type connections where you feel misunderstood, judged, alone against the team. Abandoned people often suffer from conditions that stem from the base. Also, there can be problems because you feel responsible for your family or other tribal connection. This is where it impacts on you when you are staying in a situation where you do not want to be but you are *responsible*. The marriage, the job, parenting the unwanted child, giving up the top bunk – anything where you feel responsible to mend, fix or otherwise repair a situation.

In life today, because so many people spend so much time at work, family/tribe can mean work connections or other close social cluster connections. If you are an alcoholic, if you steal things, if you have obsessive compulsive disorder, or suffer from bedwetting you have fear issues, authority issues, it shows you are struggling with your family.

Loyalty, honor and justice are key issues for the base. These are all components of responsibility. If you feel loyal and you don't want to be, or if you feel that you were owed loyalty and it was not delivered, you will run into difficulties. From circumstances as seemingly simple as being rejected for having head lice, problems can arise in the base chakra. Anything that disconnects you from your group tribe will interfere. Honor can often interfere in a much deeper way.

Base Chakra case studies:

Base Client One: Aged 56 – explosives engineer –
Problem: unexplained sore legs

Ronald was sitting in the waiting room when I came out of my clinic room to collect him.

"Hello," I smiled at him, holding out my hand, "I'm Carmel Bell."

"Hello, I'm Ronald." Ronald smiled back as he struggled to his feet. It was obvious that he was in some pain from his legs or feet.

I waited patiently for him to reach me then we shook hands before I led the way back down the hallway to my clinic room. When Ronald was seated in the comfortable armchair I have people sitting in, I took the forms he had filled in with his details on there from him and sat down opposite him to start our session.

Ronald was 56-years-old, short, stocky but mostly healthy. He had come to see me because he was having pain in his legs for no known reason. There was no muscle cramping, no arthritis and his hips were fine. Ronald liked to walk, ride pushbikes, sail and explore nature. Yet this was now being impeded by this vague aching in his legs all the time. Sometimes the pain would wake him at night.

I looked at Ronald energetically, seeing him both in my mind and in person. What I could see was a poison in Ronald's body that was in his legs, causing the pain. This was odd. Both legs, being poisoned? Ronald wanted to run away from his life, but his legs would not let him.

I started to ask questions about his life particularly family because if the pain was in the legs, then it was to do with the base chakra. Whilst I did this, I watched Ronald's energy to see what was changing. We talked about his birth family, his children, his work and his hobbies, all the clusters that would have the most significant impact on Ronald's base chakra and legs. Whilst questioning him I noticed quite a lot of heart involvement. I could see that Ronald also had high blood pressure and that it needed attention, although he told me it had not yet been diagnosed.

I kept asking questions, just talking pleasantly, until I found what I knew was the problem. Ronald had been bitten on the left leg by a sand fly about 12 months before and by a spider on the right leg around six months ago. There was poison in both legs causing muscle pain. When questioned he showed me both bite sites. Both were still inflamed and although small in size, both were still angry and tender.

Ronald's family had also been a problem for Ronald. One of his siblings blamed Ronald for their mother's death and Ronald's father, also dead, had never made Ronald feel wanted. Now Ronald was also unsure if the children he and his wife were raising were his.

Ronald's problem was that he did not feel secure with where he was in his family group, either birth or marriage group. He did not feel that he could trust any of the women around him. Both major women in his life had inflicted on him dire issues of loyalty and honor and Ronald had no idea of what he was to do. He had also felt like he could not make enough money in his profession, even though he was running his own engineering firm. In short, he felt like he was a disappointment to everyone. He was having trouble knowing what he should do with the rest of his life.

We talked about choices, we talked about obligation and we talked about what he truly wanted to do – being in France, sailing. We talked about Ronald needing to follow his own heart more. We discussed the fact that he had raised his children as if they were his, he loved them, what difference did it really make now? We talked about his needing to stay, or thinking about ending the marriage. Which path would be truer for Ronald? We talked about him not being able to change the false beliefs of others about him, with his mother's death. In the end, what difference did it make, as long as Ronald knew the truth? More to the point was why did Ronald attract women who thought the worst of him? Ronald craved peace, craved beauty, yet his profession was very male, as was his hobby. Was Ronald happy with the softer side of his nature? No, he was not, yet he wanted to be.

Ronald felt attacked and undervalued. Using the pathways through his energy system that our discussion had created, I ran Metatronic Energy through him, taught him to ground, seal and dump and then we finished.

Result: *Dear Carmel, I just wanted to thank you for seeing me last month. I thought I would update you to let you know that the insect bites are healed fully now and the pain is gone from my legs. I cannot believe what a difference it made to me. I also have had my blood pressure checked and my doctor found that I did have mild hypertension. As I do not want medication, I will try exercise first of all. My wife and I are off to France and Ireland, leaving the boys to run the house. Life is much better. Thank you for your care and understanding. Ronald*

Base Client 2: Aged 48 – aerobics instructor, life coach. Secondary Sacral

Problem: Joints, muscles, low energy. Undisclosed Lupus.

Silvana was a stunning woman whose profession was teaching people to be both fit and life wise. Her problem was she was feeling exhausted and her muscles and joints were hurting so much that it was interfering in her profession.

We sat together and started to talk. I asked the usual questions that I always begin with until I found a hit and her energy system began to alter. I could see that there was more that Silvana was not telling me with her life and conditions. I could see an autoimmune disease so I asked a few more questions. Silvana also had Lupus which would explain the joint and muscle pain, but not the low energy. Also, why did she have Lupus? Silvana was trying to ignore the Lupus and had successfully ignored it for years, but we talked about it as I could see that it was one of the physical drivers behind her ill health today. The energetic reason for developing Lupus had been ignored, so it had moved into something else. Silvana's biography was not going to disappear quietly.

Her history was she was married to a man who watched pornography obsessively. This made Silvana feel as if she was not enough for her husband. Her mother and father had faced a similar issue.

Now her three children were unhappy with Silvana staying in the marriage, yet she still loved her husband, but she felt trapped because her daughter, who was 18, was afraid of men. The daughter had been raped a few years ago. Silvana was also afraid of her own father, so she sympathized with her daughter but she was trapped in her desire to keep her marriage going and her children safe. Her cultural and religious background, both base issues, disallowed her to easily leave her husband or to disobey or refuse him. In short, Silvana was trapped, angry and frustrated.

Thus she had Lupus, an autoimmune disease and her legs were sore and tired, also from the base. And her energy was dangerously low due to the damage to the sacral chakra and her self-esteem.

Silvana was also jealous of her younger sister who was currently in the middle of a divorce so there was another huge family conflict.

I could see that if Silvana did not find peace soon the Lupus would flare up and become a real problem.

We discussed possible choices. For Silvana, divorce was not yet, and may never be, an option. Despite all, she loved her husband. The pornography was bad because they rarely had sex. They rarely had sex because she felt compared to these other women. She did not feel sexy enough for him if he also needed pornography, but he said that he needed more if she did not want to sleep with him. For people in a relationship this is almost unwinnable.

I suggested that she cut back on exercise for work and concentrate on exercise that may help her in life, like Bollywood dancing or burlesque. That she put the pornography issue aside for now and concentrate on repairing herself.

Her base chakra was damaged because she was afraid of disappointing a family group whichever way she turned. If she stayed with her husband she was upsetting her children and if she left she would upset her parents and her community. Damned if you do, damned if you don't.

Did she really need to leave? Her marriage was her problem and not her children's. They were all grown up, 18 or older, and she said that no-one had accused him of being abusive, or harmful – just distant. This was all repairable. But Silvana needed to be certain that she wanted to go, or stay, without influence from anyone.

Silvana also felt sorry for her mother and had not seen before that she was copying her mother's journey. She always thought that her mother should leave her abusive father. So Silvana just felt trapped. She wanted to give up aerobics but was afraid if she did she would not be attractive anymore to her husband and her marriage would end, so to cut back and try something new was a good suggestion.

As she was copying her mother's pattern, we needed to alter that by removing the pattern from Silvana's system. This pattern was stored in all the chakras for use as a reference. To also increase her life energy we needed to repair the sacral chakra at the same time.

I could see that by repairing the sacral and restoring her self esteem her joints and muscles would strengthen and repair. With Silvana it was more a case of too much energy stored in her system and not enough space. She was overloaded. Her diet was good, her exercise was good, she was fit and she was not struggling financially. She was struggling internally. She did not know what to do, how to proceed, what was the best. Whichever way she turned, she was sure to disappoint someone. The only sensible thing to do was to please herself.

I used Metatronic Energy to remove the patterns that were creating these issues, then I taught her how to manage the energy as it moved for herself, via dumping, grounding and sealing.

Result: Silvana let me know that she had decided to stay in her marriage. Her daughter had gone into counselling and was not being such a problem for Silvana. Her joints and muscles were greatly improved and Silvana had taken up burlesque dancing. Her energy was now normal.

Base client: aged 42 – female – accounts manager.

Fiona came to see me because she had thrush so badly, so painfully and so often that she could no longer have sex. She was also a celiac and lactose intolerant.

When we spoke about her life and her upbringing I could see that there was a huge hook in her from her mother. Whilst not uncommon, in Fiona it was enormous. As it turned out, Fiona had been born in a marriage that her mother had not wanted and all her life she had carried that guilt and that sorrow for her mother. Now, she was stuck with thrush all the time because if she had thrush she could not have guilt for having sex with her husband and enjoying sex!

She had never had children, she did not do anything that she wanted to do and she had just recently started to develop vestibulitis, which is an inflammation of the vestibular. Fiona was unhappy but trapped.

I pointed this out to her and put energy through her in the hope that it would relieve the thrush and reverse the vestibulitis.

At last report from Fiona, it had succeeded on both counts.

Exercise:

Examine what issues you may have going on in your base chakra. Are you suffering from constipation, sore legs, something else? And why? Where are you not content with your family cluster? Do you feel loved and supported by them or rejected?

Sacral Chakra –
The power of relationships and the power of Choice.

How you view you in connection to your partners.

Your personal needs and the power of union
The human level of self-esteem
The sacral chakra is located in the abdomen between umbilicus and pubic bone and is connected to the third eye.

This is your own self esteem, your ego, how you view you. Are you the kind of person who drives a Ferrari or a Mazda?

The Physiology of the Sacral Chakra

*Endocrine Gland:*Ovaries, gonads, sexual organs

Body Sections ruled by the Sacral Chakra

Hips
Large intestine
Bladder
Appendix

Prostate
Sexual organs

Mental/Emotional issues ruled by the Sacral Chakra

Personal power
Sexual issues
Financial issues
Creativity
Honor in relationships
Guilt and blame
Personal ethics
Self-confidence
Your inner self esteem
Control of relationships
Choice

Physical issues ruled by the Sacral Chakra

Gynecological problems
Bladder problems
Sexual issues (either too much or not enough)
Impotency
Fertility
Lower back pain,
Compulsive eating,
Childbirth pain,
Endometriosis,

Herpes,
Thrush,
Menopause difficulties,
Menstruation difficulties,
Prostate problems,
Premature ejaculation.

Purpose of the Sacral Chakra

To manage creative energy
Physical survival
Sex, power
Handling money
Protection of self

Fears held in the Sacral Chakra

Loss of control
Slavery
Poverty
Abandonment
Loss of the use of your body

Sacral Chakra breakdown

This is the first chakra that pulls you away from the collective. It is in here that you begin to be free to make your own choices. But that can be frightening, making your own choices. It is much easier to have someone who can tell you what to do and how it will all work out. It is much easier to rely on the collective mores' of the base chakra.

The real issue with choice is that it so often goes wrong and leaves you responsible, thus you are pulled back and forth between the base and the sacral. Just when you think you have it all worked out, it all goes wrong again.

The real lesson with the sacral chakra is to learn that we are never in control, that whatever choice we make, it will have consequences unforeseen. Order and chaos are part of the same coin. Our task is to master the chaos we feel when we lose control of the outer world. To control our responses to our emotions, just as we master our physical bodies.

It is your ability to choose your *response*, to make the best choice, that makes you a human and that gives you the power of creativity. It is through the sacral chakra that we have access to the ultimate physical creation – having children. Even men have children. But children are the ultimate cause of chaos.

In response to the chaos we feel inside, people often make poor choices. Life is chaos. Every time you think you have it worked out, something will arise to make it go wrong. You can never keep everybody and everything safe. Life is change. Growth is chaos. This tribulation will cause many problems in the sacral chakra, which is why so many people have so many sexual dysfunctions and lower back pain. When your choices are challenged or you feel as if you have been foolish, your self esteem gets challenged. You will always feel insecure when you are trying to exert control over your life.

I have seen a surprisingly high amount of businessmen who are successful – ridiculously successful – who struggle with impotence. Is it because they struggle to maintain an erection that they go into business? Or is it the business that destroys their libido?

Sacral chakra issues are all around us. It is based on your self image and that image has everything to do with sex. Wanting to look sexually attractive or wanting to look unattractive. Both are an imbalance. Sex is one of the ultimate ways of controlling another person. By withholding sex, purchasing sex, being wealthy enough or famous enough that anyone would sleep with you, you exert control over you and your life.

Sacral dysfunctions such as endometriosis are treated energetically the same way that impotence is, or herpes is, or thrush, or lower back pain. All these are issues of self esteem, self belief, creativity, sufficient money and life interest.

If you suffer from something within the sacral chakra, first look to how you feel about yourself.

It is not about the choices you make, because every choice, no matter how well intentioned it is, is capable of going wrong. Life and the energy involved are about the reason *why* you made the choice you made. You need to seek the reasons behind your choices, your motivation, and your inspiration.

Sacral Chakra case study:

Rose had cervical cancer, now she was facing six weeks of radio/chemo therapy, after undergoing a radical hysterectomy. Her life energy was low which meant that she would struggle throughout treatment, and her sacral chakra was not functioning very well. Her prognosis was poor as her cancer had been so advanced and aggressive. Rose was scared.

Rose was single now; her husband had left her but he had left her with a home, yet she felt as if she was prostituting herself to him because, although he was no longer there, it was still his home and despite his new partner, he felt he could come and go as he pleased. They had two children together, so Rose did not feel that she could tell him to stop treating her as his wife.

In short, Rose felt used and abused and trapped. She also had back problems which we traced back to a feeling that she was abandoned by her family. Now she judged that if she stood up to her ex-husband it may make her children angry with her. How was she going to have enough resilience to overcome her illness?

This was a lot of stress to be carrying whilst trying to overcome cancer.

Rose and I talked about what she wanted and the choices were available to her. I was not going to make any suggestions as to the best course of action – that was for Rose to decide. Instead I listened and whilst we talked I trickled Metatronic Energy into her body. I let the pathways between chakras lead the way into her body, then I asked her to process any thought, feeling or memory that came to her in response to her choices. She needed to feel as if she was capable of choosing a happy life, without her ex-husband. She was his equal, not his partner and not his child.

Rose and I had a few more sessions together in a short space of time as she was so unwell and needing urgent results. .

Result: Rose was a writer but she did not believe in her ability. As a result of our sessions she booked an overseas trip and was heading off to write. She had come to a new arrangement with her ex-husband that meant he was taking more responsibility for their children and giving Rose more freedom.

Her cancer was now in remission.

Sacral Case 2 – Patsy 43-year-old Client who was pregnant with an IVF assisted pregnancy and who came in for a check-up.

My client, Patsy, came to see me because she wanted a general checkup. She was over five months pregnant with a very special baby, IVF assisted after much drama and her first child.

The first thing I noted that concerned me when I looked at Patsy was a strange growth in her uterus. I was concerned. It did not look cancerous, just dangerous because it was so big. I could also see the baby – a girl – but the baby would soon not be okay if the growth continued on.

I told Patsy what I could see and asked her to go to her obstetrician for an ultrasound.

Patsy came from an English immigrant family and she felt a lack of support. Her husband was older than her and Patsy was a second wife. He had not wanted children, but she had so they had used IVF and Patsy had got pregnant. She felt on her own, even giving up work to have this baby. Pasty was none too happy to be told that I spotted a problem. She was pleased with me, but scared about the result.

Patsy rang me to thank me after she saw her obstetrician, about a month later. She told me that they had found a growth in her uterus that was likely to have killed her baby if it had not been found as the growth was growing as well. Patsy had to have surgery to remove the growth and save the life of her baby but both were okay now.

Exercise:

Are you content with your level of abundance?

Are you relying on someone else to earn for you, or tell you how much you are worth?

Do you have enough energy to live? If not, examine your self esteem. Anytime you rely on someone else to dictate your value, you will lose energy.

Solar Plexus Chakra – Identity – Personal Power

The human level of personal power

The solar plexus is located mid navel between sternum and umbilicus and links to the throat chakra.

This is the chakra that is about the most affected by how and what other people think of us. This chakra keeps us connected to the world. If you feel that the world does not like you, you will probably end up with problems somewhere here.

Physiology of the Solar Plexus Chakra

> *Endocrine Gland:* **Pancreas**
> **Body Sections ruled by the Solar Plexus Chakra**
> Kidneys Upper intestines
> Spleen
> Liver
> Gallbladder Stomach
> Mid thoracic spine

Mental/Emotional issues ruled by the Solar Plexus Chakra

> Personal honor

- Self-truth
- Sense of fear
- Courage
- Self esteem
- Confidence
- Self love
- Emotional/mental sensitivity
- Psychic sensitivity
- Assertion
- Responsibility

Physical issues ruled by the Solar Plexus Chakra

- Hepatitis
- Intestinal problems
- Irritable bowel syndrome
- Anorexia
- Vomiting
- Bulimia
- Stomach ulcers
- Hernia
- Adrenal dysfunction
- Alcoholism
- Flatulence
- Hiccoughs
- Hypoglycaemia
- Indigestion
- Motion sickness
- Morning sickness

Shingles
Jaundice

Spiritual Purpose of the Solar Plexus Chakra

Self esteem
Action
Courage
Generosity
Compassion

Fears held within the Solar Plexus Chakra

Rejection
Looking foolish
Criticism
Responsibility
Fear of unattractiveness

The Solar Breakdown

The solar plexus ties you in to humanity. You cannot escape it. If you are feeling judgmental, harsh, critical, stubborn, angered, guilty, ashamed and wanting things your own way, look out because you are destined to wind up with irritable bowel, indigestion, hepatitis or one of the other dysfunctions listed.

Most people who come to see me have an abundance of issues in their stomach or in their bowels, from worms, to hernias and flatulence. These issues are there because they are sitting in judgment of other people and also because they are feeling judged. We always expect people to behave in the way that we do. We judge others by our own responses.

The world obesity problem is a burgeoning problem nowadays. We are living in a world of people who are constantly measuring themselves against others. We are living in a world of people who want to be the best but don't want to be outstanding. People who are so angry that there is now fear everywhere about going out on public transport. But you don't need to be obese to have issues in the solar plexus. You can also be quite thin as is an anorexic, or a bulimic person.

Solar Plexus:

Age: 31 Occupation: Manager of a pharmaceutical company.

Susan was thin, but not too bony, perfect in her appearance. Her hair was neat and her clothes were impeccable. Every inch of her demonstrated carefully disciplined perfection. She looked untouchable – she was very like Grace Kelly with dark hair.

When I asked her what her reason for coming to see me was, I waited and watched her energy system with interest. The answers that people give to me are often not the reason that they are here.

Susan had an alcohol problem, she said. I could see that she did have, but I could also see much more than that. I could see that she was a bulimic but I waited before I planned to challenge her gently.

We talked about her life – how she was single in Australia but had a partner who lived overseas with his wife and children, coming to visit her every few months. This man kept telling her that he would leave his wife and son.

Susan was buying her own home and had her mother living with her. She and her mother did not get along, but Susan felt responsible for her mother. Yet Susan was very successful. She did not need to live with her mother; she did not need to have a lover overseas. She could have chosen to be happy.

She was an only child whose father had abandoned his family and whose mother had had a breakdown as a result. Susan's father was also successful and judged by Susan's mother to be a selfish and cold man.

Susan felt obligated and responsible for her mother but she felt terrible every time she succeeded and was more like her father. She felt powerless but she could not reconcile her business success with her personal failures. She was punishing her body by not allowing it nutrition.

"Do you purge, Susan?" I asked her gently. She looked truly shocked for a second and then I could see her shoulders drop.

"Yes," she nodded, "I do." It was a relief to tell someone at last.

"That's the real problem. You are feeling weak and tired because you are purging more…"

"I have to be so careful!" She exclaimed. "If I vomit too much, I lose too much weight." We smiled at each other. Susan was smart; she just needed to become comfortable with disappointing her mother by being a lot like her father.

"Iron deficient, magnesium deficient and far too much adrenaline in your system also. You suffer from panic as well?" I asked "Your adrenals are overworking."

Susan slumped. She sunk further down into her chair and nodded.

"What do you want to do about it?" I asked her. "You have a choice here, Susan. You can move ahead as you are and you will get sicker and sicker, you'll probably also out on weight despite your purging because of the hormones. Or you can change."

"Tell me what to do?" Susan asked.

"Get a separate place for your mother, lose your boyfriend and think about a relationship with someone single…" Susan nodded at all my suggestions. I knew she would never follow through. Susan was too unhappy with being successful. She could not find the balance between being her parent's child and being her own person. Her solar plexus was definitely working over time.

Even so, I taught her how to look after herself and I ran Metatronic Energy through her. Susan was caught between who she was and who she thought she should be. The more successful she was, the more her mother berated her and the more her father loved her. They hated each other and Susan was the battle ground. Until she decides to make her own decisions and live her own life, she will drink and she will purge.

Result: I saw Susan for another session after our appointment. She had moved her mother into a separate home and she said that she was feeling a lot better, but she was still drinking and purging and her boyfriend was due to visit her soon.

Choice is the most basic of all human responses. No matter what happens to us, we have the power to choose how to feel, how we respond and how we wish to proceed. Every moment is full of choice.

Susan had chosen to be a personal victim and a professional winner. I think that given enough time and a little motivation, she will be fine.

Client – 14-years-old – male – hiccoughs and anxiety/depression

A young man walked in the door, 14-years-old and slumping as he came down the hallway. He wore a very interesting t-shirt which indicated that maybe he had a sense of humor and as I could see that he was suffering from depression and a sense of doubt, that perhaps I could use his humor to help him.

John was on anti-depressants when what he needed was some good food, (he had an appalling diet) some physical activity and a whole lot of laughter.

John was having lots of self esteem issues. He had hiccoughs all the time because he was caring too much about what other people thought, particularly two much older brothers. Their energy was being pulled in through his solar plexus and he did not know where he fit in with them so he was constantly anxious. He had also been sent to a high school where he knew no-one and had not been able to form friendships. He had been premature and felt unwanted and overlooked by his parents, so their connection to him needed to be reinforced.

Quite simply, John did not know who he was. He knew who he thought he should be, but not what he was, what he wanted, or what he was good at. All of his opinions and thoughts were based on other people. Energetically he felt like an energy construct, something he was making up.

A little bit of energy management and John was feeling a lot better. I taught him also how to block people, ground and seal himself and how to sleep better at night.

Result: John is now going to a new school. He is learning to stand up for himself and to decide what he would like to do for himself. He is off the antidepressants and under the supervision of his doctor, is not showing any signs of depression now.

Exercise:

Think about the Solar Plexus and what it means. Are you being impacted here? Do you carry too much weight on your body?

Is your life being lived according to someone else's honor code?

Heart Chakra

Drive or ambition: Emotional Power

The heart chakra is the who, what, where, why, and how of life. The heart is the centre of all.

The heart chakra is located at the breastbone, to the right of the physical heart.

Physiology

Endocrine Gland: Thymus gland

Body Sections ruled by the Heart Chakra

Heart
Lungs
Shoulders
Arms
Breasts
Diaphragm
Circulatory system
Blood

Mental/Emotional issues ruled by the Heart Chakra

Drive
Love
Hope
Trust
Grief
Anger
Hatred
Loneliness
Commitment
Resentment
Self-feelings
Forgiveness
Compassion
Emotional burdens
Trust

Physical issues ruled by the Heart Chakra

Heart disease
Lung disease
Breast disease
Upper back pain/injury
Shoulder pain/injury
Allergies
Asthma
Bronchial diseases
Pneumonia

Diabetes
Anemia
A.I.D.S
Breasts too large, or too small
Hypertension
Toxins in blood and lymph system

Spiritual Purpose of the Heart Chakra

To love oneself and others
To heal
To see beauty within and without
Dedication

Fears held within the Heart Chakra

Fear of loneliness
Fear of commitment
Jealousy
Hatred
Bitterness
Anger
Inability to forgive

Heart Chakra Breakdown

The heart chakra is the centre on which we all turn and grow. Every dysfunction will take place to some degree in the heart chakra. We all feel emotional about something, sometime, somehow.

Every emotion passes through the heart and these emotions will affect all of your body. Think about it. The heart chakra is both your blood and your immune system.

You will have feelings about your illness and you will feel about how other people feel about you because you are ill, from wanting them to take care of you, to possibly feeling ashamed.

The next three chakras all belong to the upper realms of the energy system, the spiritual section. The first three are physical, humanity, whilst the heart is both spiritual and physical.

Heart Chakra

I remember a little sign in my parent's kitchen from when I was growing up that said 'Anger is one letter away from Danger.' Over the past 30 years I have thought of that often, but sadly rarely when I was angry.

Of all the emotions that humans feel, anger is about the most destructive because it has power, energy and drive. It gives you superhuman strength, and takes away most of your common sense. It destroys bodies utterly, decimates relationships and murders people in their sleep. If anger were a living human it would be residing in jail.

Carmel Bell

Angela came to see me because she was angry, but she did not know that she was angry. She thought she just had breast cancer. She had to have both her breasts removed because of an aggressive cancer and she was now having radiotherapy, but she was still not in the clear. She was feeling unwell and scared and angry. She said she did not feel feminine anymore. Her husband had become distant from her, and he had already lost her beautiful big home through his inept business dealings in which he had refused to include her in the decision making process of. All Angela had to do was sign the paperwork, which she did, trusting her husband until she had to leave the home.

Angela was angry.

She was also having an affair with a man who was not ambitious at all, probably not as powerful or successful like her husband had been but this man was gentle with her. It was whilst she was having the affair that she discovered she had cancer. She had tried to split up with her lover but found she could not. Angela was having a hard time. She felt obligated to the marriage because of what she had done, without question at first. She also had a daughter with her husband and her family relied on her husband for support and advice, which meant that Angela had to keep his failings to herself.

Now Angela was getting sicker and she was getting scared. She thought that having both her breasts cut off would mean that she was in the clear, but the cancer was spreading into her right lung and her naturopath had sent her to me. Angela had also asked her oncologist if seeing me was a good idea and had been given the all clear.

The first thing that I noticed when I looked at Angela was the anger and fear she was experiencing, then as we talked I noted how she was distant from her husband and yet not willing to leave him. I queried her about this and the affair was revealed, so now she was angry with him and herself both. Whichever way Angela turned she felt like she was cheating on someone, hurting someone, about to lose everything and she had to face this serious illness without her husband's full support.

Why was Angela giving herself such a hard time? We talked further and it transpired that her daughter had been sexually abused four years earlier, about the time that Angela would have developed the breast cancer. Just before the diagnosis actually. Angela blamed herself and her husband. They had been away at the time without their daughter, their daughter was abused and this was the result.

Her husband failed to protect them and her right breast became diseased. Now he had failed again and their house was gone. Their daughter would have to leave her prestigious private school and go to a state school. Angela had found another lover who was not as impressive as her husband, but having sex with the lover meant she was not having sex with her husband.

Angela was dying.

We talked for a while, she and I, and I pointed out to her that she was hurting no-one but herself. That if she did not love her husband she would have left him as there was no money left. Angela agreed and we dug a bit more. I explained to her that the breast cancer had occurred because she was holding anger against males in her body. We talked about her father who was deceased and how she had felt disregarded by her dad. He loved the sons and tolerated his daughters. Angela could let all this go, I explained. Once the anger energy was removed from her body along with the energy from the situations that had caused it, she would be able to heal and to send out a new and healthier signal to the Universe. This would give her more choice about how to behave and how to live her life.

Then I began the healing. It takes only a few minutes to call the energy and to run it through a system. Metatronic Energy will tend to find its own way and do as instructed through the discussion.

I called Metatronic Energy into her, with the instruction to remove the anger held against males and to replace it with compassion.

When I was done running Metatronic Energy into her a few minutes later we finished the session.

Result: For three years Angela has been a client and she remains cancer free. She is a regular client, coming about once a year for a check-up. Her affair ended not long after our session and she and her husband were able to rebuild their relationship, buy another home and earn sufficient income to allow their daughter to go back to her usual school.

Exercise:

What are your emotions telling you? Are you emotionally content, happy, satisfied or are you fooling yourself?

Are you pretending to be something you are not?

Throat Chakra

Relating to humanity   Will power

The Throat Chakra rules our highest level of communication and self-control. The Throat Chakra is located over the Thyroid Gland, in the middle of the Throat, and links to Solar Plexus Chakra

Gland: Thyroid / Parathyroid gland

Body Sections ruled by the Throat Chakra

- Throat
- Mouth
- Teeth
- Gums
- Tongue
- Trachea
- Cervical Vertebrae

Mental/Emotional issues dealt with by the Throat Chakra

- Communication
- Personal Expression
- Strength of will
- Decision-making

When All Else Fails

   Faith
   Knowledge
   Choice
   Creation

Physical dysfunctions dealt with by the Throat Chakra

   Sore throat
   Mouth ulcers
   Swollen glands
   Thyroid disease
   Gum disease
   TMJ disorder
   Whiplash
   Laryngitis
   Tonsillitis
   Oral cancer
   Tongue disorders
   Choking

Spiritual Purpose of the Throat Chakra

   Self-evaluation
   Discernment of truth
   Feeling adequate
   Open to the ideas of others
   Ability to learn from experience

Fears held within the Throat Chakra

Addictions
Criticism
Judgement
Fear of powerlessness
Fear of making money
Fear of losing control

If you consider all the things that you are afraid of, that people are afraid of, is it any surprise that people frequently have sore throats, laryngitis, pharyngitis, tonsillitis, or TMJ? The number of people who are grinding their teeth at night, whilst they sleep is concerning; because they damage their teeth, their jaw, their necks, wind up with headaches and more.

Most people are afraid of speaking out about how they really feel, whether they are feeling good or bad, nowadays. We have become a society where we are all so concerned with being 'politically' correct that no one will speak the truth. Having your opinion known and heard is frightening.

Many Autism spectrum disorder people have a lot of the dysfunctions that are listed in the throat chakra.

Throat client:
Age 39   Occupation Nurse

Sally was a thin woman, nervous and high strung. I first sensed in her that her thyroid was currently running slightly hyperactive and I knew that she would get rushes of energy through her body over the day, but that this was starting to come to an end. Sally was starting to feel her thyroid slowing down, even if no blood test was yet going to detect this.

As we talked and I questioned her further about her life, it became obvious that she had a few problems with the male energy. Her father was a fun loving guy who lived in another state and her partner had left her also, recently. Sally was afraid that she would never feel safe. She had come to see me because she was not able to get her body to feel stable. No one had been able to pinpoint the problem with her and she was at her wits end as it was now interfering with her work. She was exhausted but her fast running thyroid would not let her feel exhausted.

I explained to Sally how her thyroid was playing up and as it progressed how she would have energy surges, which she agreed she was already experiencing. The real problem was that Sally did not feel confident in any male to trust them enough to talk to them. She kept her opinions to herself and relied on no-one. Her thyroid was bearing the brunt of this and would eventually go into hashimotos disease. She would start to feel hot when she was cold; her weight would become erratic as would her energy levels. She would put on weight and her blood pressure would increase. The real problem is that hashimotos tends to cause emotional problems, which Sally was already primed for, given her history.

If we removed the signal that told her body that she could not rely on any male, she would be able to connect with someone, have a relationship and possibly and turn this around. She would feel confident enough to speak as she needed to.

Sally came in for three sessions. When she last emailed, she was doing well and two years later her energy levels were still normal. Although she was still single, she was happy.

Client: Rosemary Undiagnosed Asperger

Rosemary came to see me because she was angry about her life. Her husband was dying and was much older than she was and she felt trapped to him but loyal to him. She had no other friends, felt disconnected and could not really see much fun in her life.

She was a thin, shapeless woman, with thin grey hair in a crew cut on her head. Her clothes were grey and khaki and she was totally lacking in colour, except for her handbag which was beautiful burgundy tooled leather.

Rosemary was angry, tense, anxious and frustrated.

"Do you realize that you are an Asperger?" I asked her.

Rosemary stared at me blankly and then she blinked. "What's that?" She asked.

I explained. With each word I could see her energy and her body lifting. "This is me!" She asserted happily. I gave her the number of a service that performs assessments and also the Autism society number.

Rosemary is doing well in her new life. She now understands that she thinks and acts differently to most people and that she needs her own space and time. Rosemary is happy.

Exercise:

I would like you to consider if you are balanced, or not in your responses to life and what it throws at you. The throat is your communication chakra. Are you representing you, or someone else?

Third Eye Chakra

Outflow   Mind Power

The Third Eye Chakra rules our highest level of self-esteem.

It is located in the centre of the forehead, above and between the eyebrows.

Physiology of the Third Eye Chakra

Gland: Pituitary

Body Sections ruled by the Third Eye Chakra

Lower brain
Eyes
Nose
Ears
Nervous system

Mental/Emotional issues dealt with by the Third Eye Chakra

Intellectual intelligence

Emotional intelligence
Self-evaluation
Truth
Mastery of self
Perception of life
Openness to others views
Ability to utilize and integrate experiences
Feelings of inadequacy
Control of reactions
Logical thought
Intuitive thought

Physical dysfunctions dealt with by the Third Eye Chakra

Learning disabilities
ADD, ADHD, ASPERGERS, TOURETTES, AUTISM
Blindness
Deafness
Seizures
Anxiety disorder
Uncontrolled aggression
Neurological disturbances
Brain disorders
Tumors, strokes
Headaches
Greying hair
Balding
Memory loss

Epilepsy
Multiple sclerosis
Cold sores
Earaches
Sinus
Alzheimer's
Wrinkles
Yawning
Tiredness and waking unrefreshed
Pituitary driven Cushings disease

Fears held within the Third Eye Chakra

Afraid to see the spiritual planes
Afraid to take risks
Inability to connect with others pain
Afraid to look within self
Afraid to trust others help

Spiritual Purpose of the Third Eye Chakra

Ability to visualise
Clairvoyance
Clairaudience
Empathy
Sympathy
Willingness to take a risk

Breakdown of the Third Eye Chakra

Learning disabilities and anxiety are both increasing. They are increasing because of the increase in consciousness that the world is struggling to fulfill. The more that some people become conscious, the more threatened that they will feel. It is much easier when you can blame others for the trauma in your life.

Your third eye is your trust in you and others and your ability to care for yourself. If you have problems or issues with caring for you – it is all too hard, you will suffer from third eye dysfunction.

This chakra is also your intellectual capacity. Clairvoyants and university lecturers have more in common than they realize. They both work primarily from this chakra.

Client: Female 50 – single mother – Astrologer – Disability pensioner.

Francis was a smart, intelligent woman who lived more for her disability than she did for herself. She had learned as a young woman that she could receive more from being disabled than she ever could from being well.

She was on a disability pension, did not own her own home, was divorced from the father of her children and was not feeling very happy. She had depression and could not seem to beat it. She had tried the drugs, the therapy and we were back to drugs again.

Francis was an astrologer and used to make a living out of that, but now she wanted to 'be more' as she phrased it. She was better than that, smarter than that. Why had the world not noticed?

The trouble was that all of the time she spent moaning about her life and what she wanted to do, she was losing in what she could do.

Francis had not told me why she came to see me. As I looked it became apparent that she had migraines and that her right shoulder was badly damaged. She was also officially diagnosed high functioning Autism with panic/anxiety disorder and she was now addicted to her medication – xanax.

What a life. Beautiful woman, incredibly smart, but too trapped to see that she was her own worst enemy. Life is not a free ride; we all need to work at what we want to do. We talked for a while about her problems, she cried for a while about them, also.

We talked about how she thought about life and how possibly this was coming from her family background.

Then I used Metatronic Energy on her and I taught her how to ground, seal and dump the unneeded issues. Francis agreed to do this and we met again a month later.

A different woman walked through the door. She was bright, she was happy, she was in withdrawal from her meds and she was planning on starting practice again as an astrologer.

Francis had changed her mind and the way she thought and then she had changed her life.

Female aged 58 Issue: Nervous tic since she was 6 years old.

Lesley was a beautiful woman, well dressed and in advertising. She was calm, elegant and controlled. She just had this nervous tic in her face. It was not very noticeable unless she got stressed and then it would increase. Now she was here to see me, wanting to know why she had it and what she could do. In the past she had contemplated surgery to cut the nerves and drugs to calm her down. However, what she wanted was a solution.

The tic was in the right side of her face and it carried with it the signature of Tourettes. Lesley was not married. She had been but was now divorced which was a good thing, according to her. She did have one child whom she called a miracle baby because he came out of an affair and she did not have to share him. Her son was also gay, which Lesley saw as a good thing.

I could see a lot of anger towards the males in her life and I was intrigued. She had deliberately shut herself off energetically from what she saw as aggressive male energy to the point where her son was gay.

Lesley did not feel safe and when we talked about this she agreed that she did not trust anyone.

She had an ex-partner living with her, but not together which meant that she was staying single with no hope of repartnering.

I could see that each time we talked about males, male energy or anything to do with masculine issues, Lesley's auric field would shatter. Each time I caused this, her tic would increase.

So I went looking. Her father had abused her. Not long after this she had developed the tic when after she got a fever that was suspected as Polio. Lesley thought that her father's abuse had caused the tic.

At the time that she was first struck down with this fever, she was walking to see her godfather, with her mother and they had been confronted by a large, angry German shepherd. Lesley had fainted and woken up sick. I thought that the tic had originally been caused by neurological damage from the virus she contracted that happened to weaken her when she met the dog. Humanly, Lesley had been unlucky. But now, years later it was more body memory than an actual tic. Lesley was expecting me to say Tourettes, like so many other people had. I disagreed. It was a body reacting the way it had been taught to, that was all.

We talked about the story that I saw – lack of trust in men, lack of safety, needing to keep people away from her and maintaining fairly phenomenal control of her so that she could live and feel safe. The tic helped to keep her safe.

I ran Metatronic Energy through Lesley and we talked about her managing the energy for herself.

Result: At last report from Lesley, the tic was under control unless she was stressed badly. She is happy with the results.

Crown Chakra – Divine Power

Self acceptance

The crown deals with self-identity in connection with the Divine. It is also your highest level of acceptance of yourself.

Physiology of the Crown Chakra

> *Gland: Pineal*

Body Sections ruled by the Crown

> Pineal
> Muscular system
> Skeletal system
> Skin
> Upper brain
> Central Nervous system

Mental/Emotional issues handled by the Crown

> Faith

Inspiration
Selflessness
Connection to mankind
Spirituality
Trust in life process
Values, morals, ethics

Physical dysfunctions ruled by the Crown

Energetic disorders
Dark night of the soul depression
Chronic exhaustion unrelated to known physical cause
Head injuries
Spinal injuries
Extreme sensitivities to environment
Strange new fears

Spiritual Purpose of the Crown Chakra

Life purpose
Past life recall
Spiritual awakening
Human life force
Devotion
Inspiration
Nourishment
To live fully in the present moment

Fears held within the Crown Chakra

Spiritual abandonment
Loss of identity
Loss of connection to life and people

Crown Chakra breakdown

The long, dark tea time of the soul. That is what the crown chakra when it is in crisis is all about. The long, dark, tea time of the soul. A place where you sit isolated in a crowd, achievements at your feet, but nothing feeling good enough. When you are lost, so lost that you cannot believe it, you have a crown dysfunction. Don't give up.

This is the time to pull your socks up, laugh as hard as you can and seriously start looking at what you want to do with your life. Not what others want you to do, *but you.* If you are doing things you cannot stand, try to stop them. I know that it is not possible to change things all at once. We all have responsibilities and let's be honest, if you walked away from them all you might feel liberated but you will also feel lousy and that will not help your quest.

One thing at a time. Make one change at a time, and see what difference it may make.

It is possible that you are heading for a dark night. Most people on a spiritual journey will go there. Are you going to learn from it, or fight it?

Carmel Bell

Brief Crown case study

I had a client once who was the most depressed person I have ever seen. She was not crying, she was not unpleasant, there was absolutely no life in her, no joy in her. Nothing mattered to her, but trying to feel better, because she knew that how she was feeling was not normal. There was nothing extraordinary about her life. She had not been abused, she had not been divorced, she had no falling out with a group of friends and she was a teacher in the government sector, so she was job secure. But the problem was that she felt as if she had wasted every day of her life. She had done nothing and she felt she meant nothing.

I ran Metatronic Energy through her and I encouraged her to be happy with what she did have and also to get herself a dog to look after and train. A significant portion of people who are in the dark night lose all connection to that which is physical. Every living creature needs to be touched. Her dog was a life saver.

Crown Case study:
Male – 50's - Psychic Development teacher
Issue – Unknown virus, complete exhaustion

Albert was a psychic development teacher and a successful one at that, but this meant that when he was in crisis he did not want other people to know. The trouble with Albert is that he had lost his wife 11 years ago and he was lonely and mad. He had helped God, he thought, so why did God take it away from him?

Now he had an unknown virus and his eyes were sore, his liver inflamed, his spleen was tender and his kidneys were over functioning. His energy was really stagnant. He slept but never felt refreshed.

But what brought him to me was that he was now developing allergies.

This was a man who had spent his life trying to help spirit and he felt abandoned and betrayed. He did not feel depressed because he was not classically depressed. He was not crying a lot, going without or anything. He was living his life and he was doing the best he could. It is just that he was feeling more and more like a fraud because he did not believe that the world or Heaven made sense anymore.

I pointed out to Albert that he was depressed, suffering from the long dark night of the soul. We talked about what this meant and that it was actually normal for him, having been such a spiritual pioneer, to have reached a point of disillusionment.

Now he needed to learn to trust again and learn that if even if he cannot see the sense, there is sense there. If he could do that, life would improve rapidly.

I ran Metatronic Energy through him, gave him some exercises that he could do and we finished our session.

As usual I asked him to email me if he had anything he would like to report.

Dear Carmel,
I saw you for a session about six weeks ago. Thank you for seeing me. I'll be honest and say I did not expect the results I got. What you told me

seemed too simple, and it seemed that I should have known it myself. I think I needed to hear it from somebody else.

I am feeling much better. I sleep better and my energy is almost normal again. I am not in any pain and I hope that this continues! I know that I still have a long way to go, but I think I can make it now.

Kind regards,
Albert

Chapter Thirteen:

Self Healing

Healing may not be so much about getting better, as about letting go of everything that isn't you - all of the expectations, all of the beliefs - and becoming who you are.
-- Rachel Naomi Remen

What does healing mean? I don't know what it means for you but for me it means getting rid of what is annoying me.

Like brain damage. It was annoying me and now it is gone. Here today, gone tomorrow. It was just gone because I knew that it could be. I did not like brain damage. I cannot explain in this book how awful brain damage feels. I am happy to see it gone.

And you may notice my use of the word 'knew'. I did not 'believe' I could rid myself of brain damage, I knew. And I trusted.

What do you need to get rid of?

A healing on yourself.

This is what we are going to do. We are going to think about what the problem is so that you can lay pathways in to your energy system.

This is simple to do, by just thinking through the issue. Nothing too arduous.

- My problem is..............................(fill in the blank. This may be a sore back, headaches, or irritable bowel syndrome. Anything that is troubling you.)
- When I think about this problem, this (blank) image comes to mind straight away. Write down whatever it is. For instance that may be a song, an event, a day, a feeling, a person, a book or all of those things. You may think of several things.
- Can I feel that (problem/image) in my body somewhere? Yes, or no.

Question for you.

Have you looked up the major chakra that is connected to your current dilemma? Such as constant earaches, which would be in the third eye chakra.

You have a healing from someone, or take antibiotics, or even do both, and relieve your aching ears. Then the next week you come down with sinus infection, or sudden onset of anxiety. Once these issues are relieved you notice that your hair is starting to go grey - rapidly.

This is why, although it is very handy to know why you may have a specific illness, you need to empty the chakra of anything that is connected with an imbalance in the whole chakra, not just in connection with one disorder. Having an illness in the chakra indicates that all the chakra is in imbalance and is overloaded.

And you also need to realize that it is not just negative experiences that create blocks, it is everything, whether you view that experience as positive or negative. Whatever takes you away from right here, right now, weakens you.

So remember – you are not healing that one disorder. You are healing the entire chakra because if you do not, the dysfunction will move from one illness to another. Toothache to sore jaw, to sore throat, to sinus problems. Same problem, different disorder.

Now you are going to call in Metatronic Energy to you.

As before, hold out your right hand. We hold out the right hand because the right hand pushes, the left hand pulls. This ensures that this Energy will not go into you, until you want it to. Another reason why so many healers get so sick so quickly is because they give away their energy to others, and they absorb back into themselves the issues that was making their client unwell. This is lovely for your client, but not healthy for you.

You can do this, without becoming ill. Who has had enough of being the wounded healer? If you have, remember that Energy does not need to circulate through you to go to another person. You also do not need to bring anything of theirs into you.

So here we are, together, grounded and sealed. We have laid our pathway in through the chakra system and then we call Metatronic Energy in.

Hold out your right hand.

Ask Metatron to deliver the energy to you. Look for that same feeling that you had before – cool, light and sparkling. Not heavy, not consistent, just light.

Wait until you feel it. Cool, sparkling, light and shining.

When you can feel the light sparkle of Metatronic energy on your hand, raise your hand over your head and drop the Metatronic Energy onto your crown chakra.

The Metatronic Energy will move down into your body. You will feel a slight shiver as it passes through each chakra.

Seal yourself again in gold energy

You are done.

This is not how we do a healing on another person, but it is the most effective way to do one on you. You cannot easily feel Metatronic Energy on your own body but you can feel it on the inside of you, through your chakra system, and you will know when to stop dropping energy in. You will find that you really do only need to run energy for a few minutes.

There are some protocols to go through post healing.

General information for after your session:

It takes 24 hours for the Metatronic® Energy work to complete its cycle through your energy system, however the results and the energy release will continue for many weeks. We have set up healing in this way so that you will receive a sustained and consistent healing, rather than one big 'hit' to your energy system. You may feel many different energy shifts through your system as a result of this work. You may also experience one or more responses to this energy work.

You will notice that you get energy releases in clusters – a lot in one or a few days and then nothing for a few days, and then more again and on it will go. The more you GROUND, SEAL and RELEASE the longer the Energy will flow for you.

Responses to the Metatronic Energy Work

The two most common <u>emotional</u> reactions to a healing of this level are:
- To feel increasingly better as the old, unwanted energy is released.
- To feel an emotional reaction and perhaps even feel the need to cry. Some people feel quite down for around 72 hours. (three days) If you fall into this category you will feel much better in three days.

Both reactions are completely normal and should be viewed as a positive response.

Any emotional reaction can be expected to continue for around 72 hours. After that time you will find that the reaction suddenly stops and if you were feeling down, you will suddenly feel much more balanced.

You are likely to find that you also experience a renewed sense of hope/optimism.

<u>Physical</u> responses vary from person to person. The more common reported reactions are:
- A release of toxins via excretion and urination. Please drink more fluids (water) to hasten this process. I would like you to drink 2 litres of good quality water per day.
- A diminishing and/or alteration of physical pain and symptoms. Sometimes your physical symptoms may increase for a short duration of time. In this event do not worry – they will ease again.

To maintain your <u>physical</u> and <u>emotional</u> healing for the longest time possible, it is advisable for you to GROUND and SEAL your energy system each day, or as often as necessary to maintain your balance. It is possible for you to UNGROUND as soon as you GROUND. Sometimes you may need to ground several times in a row.

It is also possible for you to become unsealed immediately.

<u>The Spiritual Release:</u> For the next 72 hours you will be releasing a lot of unwanted energy that was at-

tached to issues that you have truly dealt with and these issues will be moving out of your energy system. View this as 'dusting the shelves'. You will most likely find that you have a lot of "Aha!" reactions as you remember events that you had forgotten, or even thought that you had already released through other methods. This releasing is the final stage, where the 'splinters' are removed from the system. Metatronic® Energy is specifically designed for this level of release. You will retain the memory of the incident(s), but not the emotional / spiritual toxins that continued to call the same lessons to you. Try not to analyze, or think too much about what you are feeling/seeing/remembering: simply let it go. Even if you feel emotionally attached, please remember to release. This is most easily done through gratitude for the lesson taught by that experience and by tossing into your energy bin.

Post 72 hours

After 72 hours, issues that you have not finished with will be able to move up into your consciousness to be dealt with. These are issues that have not yet been processed fully and may require further energy release. It is quite common for symptoms to alter as what was hidden will now be revealed by the release work you have done. In other words, if there was an underlying pathology being hidden by your current dysfunction, this can often be revealed so that you can discover what the real problem is. This may be a physical or emotional dysfunction.

How long will the healing last for?

These are AVERAGES. Often a healing will last indefinitely.

1st session on an average of six weeks

2nd session on an average of eight weeks

3rd session – indefinite length of time. This may be as little as a week or as long as a year or more.

Basically it depends on how well you do your 'work'.

For less chronic conditions most people find that one or two Healings are enough to achieve their desired results.

Each time you receive Metatronic® level Healing, and release more issues you get a more sustained result.

What next?
- You've learnt to Ground (small red circle). You've learnt to Seal (Gold liquid). What next?
- Next we DUMP or THROW INTO THE BIN what has been holding us back, and then we choose to feel another way.
- Four very simple steps.
- You are not trying to eliminate the moments that caused you problems. You are trying to release the pattern of the energy. Don't be concerned with what arises. Just release it and move on

with your day. Be amazed with the things that occur in your life as a result.

Exercise Seven : Throwing Into The Bin or dumping

Why do we do this? You need to signal to your energy system that you are no longer willing to keep the old energy within your body. This is best done with the ***clear intent*** of throwing out anything that you no longer need. These energies may from either positive or negative experiences. They may be represented as physical aches and pains as well and not just memories or dreams or thoughts.

Dumping: Imagine, see or feel a small rubbish bin next to you. This bin will stay with you for as long as you need it. It will empty automatically. You can do the physical action of tossing, or you can do it mentally as well. Anything that arises, be it a thought, feeling, dream or memory, or even a physical ache or pain – throw into your bin. Just pretend that you are grabbing it, from wherever you may be feeling it and then throw this into your energy bin. The more you discard, the better you will get. Your body will alter in response to this discarding of unwanted energy.

<u>Choose to feel another way. Make a better choice.</u>

Whatever you have removed, choose to replace it with something more positive. Choose to feel happy or content. No one can tell you how to feel. Every emotion, whether we see that emotion as good or bad, is an acceptable emotion. Acknowledge it then make a better choice as to how you will react, respond, feel.

And this above all things remember – to thine own self be true.

1. Ground
2. Seal
3. Throw into the Bin
4. Choose to feel another way

Section Two:

Dying and Living

Chapter fourteen:

Meetings with Metatron

July 1966

I am burning and I am running. I can feel the flames ripping through the skin on my legs, eating the nightgown from around my body and melting through the scarf tied around my head. I feel a tightening around my neck and I gasp. The air is hot, burning inside my lungs.

I can hear a roaring noise inside my head but there is no time to think about it. My brain can only record fear and pain. I can smell roasting meat.

Then I fall, tripping over my blistered feet.

Before I hit the ground I am in a passageway and there is a light.

I feel nothing for a moment, and then there is coolness around me.

I walk towards the light further down the passage. It is not a bright light, like street lights at night, but it is a soft and clear light. I am puzzled because I do not know why I am 'here'. I do not know where 'here' is. I feel like I have been on a long trip and I have just woken up. I am clearheaded but I am lost.

Suddenly, I remember burning. I remember fire dancing around me. I remember looking down when I felt pain and I remember the blue inside the orange flames licking my body and arcing up. I remember the beauty of the flames, the color and the patterns before I remember the pain of my flesh roasting, the smell, the sensation of fear, and the heat. But mostly I remember the heat.

Then running, I can remember running. I could not scream – there was no air. But now I am walking and this makes no sense.

I am four years old.

I hear a noise, like my name being called. I look back over my shoulder but there is nothing there that I can see. I feel a little nervous. It is so quiet. Up ahead I can see some vague shapes in a mist of light. I rub my eyes and keep on walking. My foot fall makes no sound.

A space opens up in front of me and I am no longer in a passage. I am in a place? There is a tree. I recognize it as a palm tree. It is large and lush and green and there are two people standing near the tree. And there are gates in front of me. I walk towards the gates, entranced. The gates are huge, towering above me and spreading out to either side, silver and alive. In the metal I see every animal I know and many more that I have never seen, mixed in with plants and trees, flowers and grasses, all together – held in these living gates.

One of the two people who had been standing by the palm tree walks towards me. He stops when he is standing next to me, on my left.

"Hello Carmel," he says. I look up at him. He looks like someone from a painting that I have seen in the church that my parents take me to, but more real than the painting. Brown hair, a beard, tanned face and white robes.

"Hello," I reply.

"You aren't meant to go any further," he says to me. I just look at him and then look back at the gates.

"Why not?" I ask finally when he says nothing more.

"Because you have a task to do," this man kneels down to talk to me. I look into his eyes and I feel good, I feel safe, I feel love. I like it here. His hair is a light brown and his eyes are blue grey, like the ocean. I have only seen the ocean a few times. I live far in the country. My father's eyes are brown, and my eyes are blue green.

"Who are you?"

"I am Jesus, your grandfather." He smiles at me.

The second man moves forward and also kneels down. He is taller than the first man, and his shoulders are wider. His hair is silver. "Hello Carmel," He says. "I am Metatron." He smiles at me also. He is harder to see. It feels slippery when I look at him. But I can see that he is also a male; I can see that he is beautiful but sometimes he has a beard and sometimes he does not. He shimmers like lightning, crackles with energy, but he feels good and safe, like the warm hand that reaches out from the dark in the middle of night when you are scared.

"Metatron," I repeat. He begins to speak to me, telling me about the world to come and my place in it. He tells me how I will help people, how I will heal people. He tells me that it will be hard and I will be hurt, but when I have taught enough, this energy would go on by itself and I could come home then, but I could not stay here now.

Metatron holds out his right hand and I place my left hand into his. His fingers curl around my hand and I can feel a tingle run up my arm into my chest. I can feel it in my heart. I can feel the tingle as it moves through me. It is the living embodiment of the energy I can see in him. It is in his hand and now it is in my hand, too.

"This is your gift, Carmel," Metatron explains. This feeling is still running through my body, as if it is on a quest. I can feel it and I wonder what it is doing. If feels as if every bit of me is filling up with this energy and then Metatron takes his hand away and stands up. "You will be a doctor but not a doctor," he explains to me. In Heaven, any thought is accompanied by a mental image and now I could see images in my mind of me talking to people, telling them about their bodies, but it was in a way that was casual, relaxed and not at all like the formal doctors that I saw when I was taken for check-ups.

"I will remember," I promise him when he finishes.

Jesus walks forward to me. "It is time," he says to Metatron and then he looks at me. His eyes are now deep blue and I start to cry. I do not want to go back.

Jesus, Metatron and a palm tree, standing on sandy ground; an oasis in a desert. 'I will remember!' I think to myself. I know so much more than has been said to me in words. I can still feel Metatron's energy running through me.

"Will anyone help me?" I am feeling weak now, tired all of a sudden.

"Your 'soul mate' will help you," I think I hear Jesus say. I am fading. The tree is growing dim.

"Who is he?" I ask urgently because I can hear a drumming sound and it feels like something is tugging me.

"Bernie..." I hear. "Your husband..."

"Bernie." I promise myself as it all goes suddenly black. It is the first time I have heard that name.

Then there is nothing but pain.

I had accidentally set myself on fire in the early hours of morning, in my parent's home. It was a cold winter's morning. Ablaze, I ran until I fell to the floor, burning and dying.

'Something' woke my father up; he is not sure what it was that woke him, except perhaps for a full bladder. My father got out of bed and went walking to the toilet when he noticed a light on, down the house. He was tempted to ignore the light when he realized that it was flickering. Running now, he found me, lying on the floor ablaze, the nylon scarf that I had tied around my head to keep my hair off my face whilst cleaning for my mother, was melting into my neck.

My father beat the flames out with his bare hands and then he wrapped me in a blanket and drove me to hospital.

I died in that fire and although I was dead for a just a few short minutes, those minutes changed my life and set me on a path, searching for a profession that was not yet known about and I had no clue of, or of where to start looking. I just knew that there was something that was calling me. I knew I could do something that I could not explain. I could still feel it in my hand and in my heart.

After I woke up in hospital, bandaged and in pain, I automatically started calling this energy to me that Metatron introduced me to. I did not think about it, it just happened.

I called the energy to my body and I let it go into me and do as it wanted. I had no idea how to direct this energy; I had no idea what this energy could do, or how long I should use it for. I just focused on the feel of it and of calling it to me until the pain would leave me and then I would forget about it until I was in pain again.

When I was released from hospital, scarred, terrified of fire and bleeding from my kidneys so that all my urine would appear pink, I let the memory of my NDE go. Apart from the name 'Metatron', I forgot about my NDE and my time in Heaven for many years.

I still knew that I wanted to be a doctor, particularly after such close encounters with so many doctors, but I knew I never would be.

The fire had burned most of my lower body, my hands and feet and some of my chest and arms. It had melted the nylon scarf into my neck. It had also damaged my kidneys and I was told that I was not likely to have children.

I would use the energy that Metatron had shown me on myself whenever I was unwell, to repair the damage to my body. I still had no clear idea of what I was doing, but I found this energy felt fantastic and it would keep me well and feeling healthy when other people around me got sick, or when I was supposed to be sick. On several occasions I was supposed to be ill with kidney problems caused by the fire but I worked on them with this energy. I now have no visible scars from the fire and no other damage.

I experimented with the Metatronic Energy every chance I got. I practiced on me, my animals and my brother and sisters. I would pretend that I was a doctor and then I would do magic to make them well. My dolls had to sit patiently for their turn to be seen and then when they were, get injections so that I could practice.

During my childhood years I noticed that I could also see energy around people and animals, plants and other objects. It looked like a heat haze or a mirage but with much clearer boundaries. I had no way of understanding what this energy I was seeing meant and there was no-one that I knew of who could help me; each time I would speak to someone about what I was seeing that would tell me that they did not know what I was talking about.

I began a quiet 'study' of my own, by watching and mentally recording the different colors and different patterns around people. After a while I realized that I *could* tell what a color or pattern meant. The same colours would mean the same dysfunction, regardless of who it was. Auras were not 'personally' chosen – they were created by what people were feeling and how well or unwell their bodies and their minds were.

I also learned that this energy around people looked different when they lied to how their aura appeared when they told the truth. My world was colourful and fascinating.

When All Else Fails

One day, when I was eleven years old, my mother took me to see a kidney specialist, after a particularly persistent attack of kidney fever, as she used to call it. It was then that I was told that if this kept happening to me and I became sicker, the option was removing one or both of my kidneys.

I was too young to remember all the details but I do remember thinking to myself – 'No. This is not going to happen to me.' When I got home I went to my room and I sat quietly by myself. I thought back to the time when this started, when I had burned. I remembered talking to Jesus and Metatron, and I remembered again the energy that Metatron had given me.

I decided then that I could fix this, that I did not need a doctor to do this for me because all that they offered was medicine and surgery. I wanted neither option.

Without knowing what I was doing, I called energy to me that I had felt in Heaven and I let this feeling run into my head. I could feel the energy running through my body. I could feel it working on my insides. I deliberately thought about how I had felt when I burned. Scared, alone, lost, unloved and abandoned. I felt powerless and afraid. I felt like my whole world and all my choices were being taken from me. I thought about all this and I ran energy through me.

I also thought about all the responsibility that I felt at home, helping my mother do chores and looking after my siblings, some of whom were younger and some older. I thought a lot about a lot, anything that made me feel powerless and trapped. All these feelings felt like this sickness to me. I could feel and see the feelings in my body. When I was reasonably sure that I knew what these feelings were, I let them all go and I thought to myself that now I was going to have fun. I had been sick long enough.

I left my room and went to find my mother. She was in the kitchen starting dinner. I walked around the bench to stand next to her.

"Mum," I spoke.

"Yes Carmel?" she responded, without looking up from her task of peeling potatoes. I took one potato away from her.

"I'm not sick anymore," I told her.

She looked at me in surprise. "How do you know?"

"I fixed it." I responded.

Mum laughed softly, "You've always been strange," she smiled.

November 1979

It was minor surgery.

When I was 17 I had met a Bernie and I had married him, even though I was so young. I loved him and I had been told that Bernie was my soul mate, but this felt wrong. I did not know why it would feel wrong. I was following the hints given to me by spirit, but I had desperately not wanted to say yes at our wedding. I was happy to be with him, just not married. Even though I loved Bernie, I was terrified.

I had left school a couple of years before when I had suddenly felt that there was no place for me at my parent's home. At 15 years old, I left school, got a job to support myself and moved out of home, ready to take on the world.

But then I needed a minor operation so here I was, sitting in hospital, waiting for my turn.

For some reason I felt nervous going into surgery. My mind wandered back to when I was four and in hospital after the fire. I thought about the NDE that I had experienced and, even though I was convinced it had happened to me I was still unsure of whom Metatron really was. Was he an angel or was I making it all up?

'Who is Metatron?' I remember I had asked my mother when I was recovering from the fire.

'An angel.' She had answered, busy with doing things. 'Why?' Mum asked.

I looked at her and shrugged. An angel. Something for the priest, then, or preferably forgotten about.

Now, years later as I am wheeled into the waiting bay for the operating theatre, where a drip was placed into my hand, I suddenly remember Metatron again. I also remember the anesthetist leaning over me, patting my hand before inserting the needle into my hand and I am surprised at how quickly a fog drifts across my eyes as cold rushes up my arm and into my chest. I am unconscious.

My next moment is filled with light and once again I find myself standing in that same place as before. It looks like the desert, and I can see the palm tree again. I see a pyramid in the distance and I realize that I am in Egypt.

There are Jesus and Metatron again, waiting for me and there are also a couple of other people standing with them.

I walk forward, confused. "Why am I here?" I ask.

"You died." Jesus states simply. I hold out my hand and look at it. It looks alive. I am confused.

"Dead?" I ask, querulously.

"Don't be concerned. You are not staying."

"We wanted to talk to you." Metatron speaks as the two other beings move forward to stand next to him.

He introduces them to me and I feel like I am in a strange kind of board meeting.

Hiram and Peter; these were my helpers, and my guides. We hold hands and with the touch, I feel memories burn into me. Hands seemed to let energy flow into your body.

Hiram was my husband in a few past lives, the last time being in Egypt and Peter has been my companion always, it seems. Now they were with me as a doctor and a priest, custom made for the job Metatron wanted me to do.

Metatron reminded me again of how I was to be using the energy he had given me, use it and pass it on.

Then Metatron continued, "You married the wrong man," he stated simply. "He is not your soul mate." I look at Metatron and I can feel an enormous sorrow fill my heart. This is going to hurt, I know it.

I hear a loud buzzing that grows until it drowns out my own heart beat. I smell something and my mouth and throat are parched.

"Water..." I croak.

When All Else Fails

A face appears above me. "Not yet," says the mouth attached to the face. "Have this." An ice block is placed into my mouth gently and my head is lifted as I suck it.

After a while I fall asleep, feeling cold and warm. Moving hurts my chest.

A little time further on and a face appears above me. It is my doctor, with a hospital cap on his head. "Am I all right?" I croak. This was minor surgery and I feel terrible.

"You're fine, Carmel, but you will have to stay in overnight. We had a slight problem…"

My heart had stopped. They had to stop the operation and restart me.

Seeing Metatron again stayed in my mind this time. Being told that I was with the wrong Bernie was devastating. I knew that I was meant to be with Bernie and I could not reconcile this predicament inside myself. I was utterly torn between wanting to stay with my husband and knowing that I was in the wrong place, with the wrong man.

So I continued on with my normal life, working and hanging out with interesting people, doing clairvoyant readings and playing with this energy on the side. I studied anything and everything to do with esoteric lore that I could find, from old books to spells that I was told about. I read about the aura and studied wicca books and more. I became an excellent clairvoyant.

I also had a little boy with Bernie, but within two years of our son's birth, our relationship had sadly ended. I became a single mother and once again I found myself using the skills I had developed to help people and support my child and me. Life moved along, feeling empty. It felt like there was something missing but I could not say what it was. I just felt like I was missing the point.

I wished that Metatron, Jesus, Peter or Hiram would just tell me what I should do and where I should head instead of maintaining silence whenever I asked questions for me.

But it seemed like doing that would be too simple, too logical. I was left alone.

My 'secret' life as a healer continued and even thrived. I was getting better and faster at using this energy that Metatron had given me, but I knew that there was something more to find, something more that needed to be added into the mix. People were getting results but I was not getting the lasting results I was hoping for. I kept searching.

July 1986

'Learn massage,' the voice whispered into my mind.

"What?" I asked out loud. "You must be mad!" I stated firmly whilst I continued with what I was doing. I was sewing a wedding dress, great swathes of white fabric – organza and satin – flowing everywhere. In between Medical Clairvoyance, as I now called it, I now ran a design and dressmaking business as I loved to sew and create and it was the continuation of a business I had started when I was 10, making Barbie clothes. I was now working under Emphasis Designs and it was doing really well. I had a few people working for me and was creating bespoke garments for people overseas as well as in Australia.

My mind drifting, I kept feeding fabric through my machine.

'Learn massage.' The voice spoke again.

"Peter?" I asked out loud.

"Peter," the voice confirmed.

"Why?" Silence. I sighed. "I should be used to this by now," I muttered when there was no further response.

A few days later when the local paper was delivered I opened it up and casually flicked through the paper when my eye fell on an ad for a massage school. It was the first time I had ever seen the ad, but feeling like a fool I rang the school and after initial enquiries, I enrolled.

Within a fortnight I was sitting in the massage school, looking at all the people coming in around me. They were mostly young people, about 18 or 19, clearly excited to be off on a new path. I felt completely out of place and I was also wondering where the models were.

I turned back to the front of the classroom and phased out, letting my mind go blank when Peter spoke to me again. "Turn around." He said. I automatically turned and looked.

In the doorway there was a small group of people who had just walked in together and in the middle off this group stood a man, chatting and laughing. He was short, had sandy blonde hair with a moustache and very broad shoulders. He looked forward suddenly, right at me and I felt my heart stop. And I knew.

There was Bernie, at last. 'Where have you been? I've been waiting.' I thought, turning back to face the front of the room.

Both of us had other commitments so we became friends. But at last, there was Bernie.

Bernie and I let each other go whilst acknowledging to each other that we loved each other. I continued on with my life, seeing clients, sewing, and being friends with Bernie. Then I discovered I was pregnant to my partner. This was definitely not planned.

Because of the pregnancy my relationship fell apart, I left my partner just weeks before we were to be married, closed my dressmaking business and moved away to have my baby on my own. I continued on with Medical Clairvoyance because that was transportable and people seemed to follow me, not matter where I went.

March 1991

I had just given birth to my second son and I was bleeding, a lot. Once again, I needed surgery and I was not looking forward to it. My infant son, James, was placed into a crib and he was wheeled away. I had given him his name, but that was all I had given him. I was crying. I felt scared and I did not know why.

My life had not gone the way I wanted it to. I was lost, alone and struggling. I had walked away from Bernie and I had lost my partner and become a single parent again. I had been working as a Medical Clairvoyant for a few years now; with good success even if no-one – not even me – understood what it was that I was doing. Even so, people kept finding me and coming to see me, though. As well, I was running another business that was more normal and socially acceptable but I had lost my relationship because of the Medical Clairvoyance, my partner preferring to think of me as insane rather than anything else. And now I was faced with having my second child and raising both children on my own.

And just to top of a perfect life, now I was facing surgery one more time.

"Look after them," I asked my sister about my sons, as I was wheeled away.

"I will," She promised. I knew she would. She was their guardian and would love them for me if I died, but I really wanted to see them both grown. I did not think I would.

In the pre-op room, "I'm scared." I tell the anesthetist.

"You'll be fine," He tells me in a disinterested way then begins his list of questions before administering his drugs. Once again the familiar rush of cold down my arm and into my chest. This time a really loud hum in my ears and the world spins uncontrollably. I am gone.

Metatron moved forward and looks at me. He says nothing and I say nothing. We look at each other. I do not know what he wants. I know I am not dead. I know I will return. In my mind I hear reassurance of that fact from Metatron. I can feel his concern for me. Life has been hard and very dark these last few years.

"There are two paths in front of you. You are free to choose which one you would like." Metatron finally says. There is no judgment in his voice, no hint of what I should do, or not do. This is the simple telling of fact. I have a choice. Heaven is letting me off the hook.

In my mind I see the two paths of which he speaks. One path will lead to an ordinary life, frustration, boredom and then death. I will love but I will not achieve anything. But I will see my sons grown.

The second path will lead through a jungle of heartache and betrayal, sorrow and isolation, but I will find the person I have been looking for. I will be loved. I will change the world.

I could scream. I could pummel Metatron with my fists. "Why!?" I am shown a man I already know, but walked away from. Years ago I was told to find Bernie and I had, but it was the wrong Bernie and then I had met another Bernie, but had walked away from a relationship with him because we were both committed to other people. Yet now I was being shown these paths. Now I was being shown that I had been wrong to walk away from him.

"You are being given a choice." Metatron tells me, with compassion.

I fall to my knees and cry. I am alone. I am in Heaven and yet I am alone. But I know which path I will choose. I have no choice.

When I am released from recovery back to my room, my baby, James, is handed to me. I am attached to a drip receiving blood to replace all that I lost. I feel terrible and weak, but I am in love with my little, unwanted, unplanned son. His enormous fists are balled up next to his cheeks and his eyes are wide open. He looks at me in such a quizzical way that I am amazed. I know he will have a hard life, I know he will face much of the rejection for me but I love him. He is mine.

I leave the hospital with my infant son and the memory of Metatron fresh in my mind a week later. I have chosen and this time there is no room for anything else.

But I have no idea where I will find Bernie.

December 1992

Life had been almost impossible this past year and a half since James was born. I had been on my own, working as a Medical Intuitive, trying to understand it what I was doing. Every time I would try to leave this profession, people would phone me, asking desperately if I could see them, or I would get a feeling, again, that this was what I needed to be doing. That feeling would haunt me until I started seeing people again. I felt damned either way.

My question was - if I was doing what Heaven wanted me to do why was it so damn hard?

My mother always used to tell me that God tested his friends most thoroughly and I used to tell her that I wished that he would not be so friendly to me.

But by 1992 people were finding me quickly and easily and there was no shortage of clients even though I never advertised. Every time I saw a client I would struggle with what I was doing and how I was doing it.

I would tell people what their illness was but then I did not know what I could do to help them, or what they should do with the information. All I could do was recommend that they see their doctor and although this seemed like sensible advice, it also seemed pointless to me. I had no training in medicine, naturopathy, or energy healing, other than my own experiments with Metatronic Energy and my scientific nature and brain wanted validation before I went widely public.

That people were referring others onto me and coming back themselves was good proof that what I was doing was helpful, but I still struggled, still I sought clarity inside me.

I remember the first time that I deliberately used Metatronic Energy on a client - a lady named Maureen. Maureen had come to see me because she was overweight and unhappy. She was suffering from depression but despite medication and counselling, she was not feeling better. Nothing seemed to help and she was miserable. She had heard of me and decided to see if I could offer anything new. Before I saw Maureen I would offer a diagnosis to people but how they dealt with the information was up to them. Now, with Maureen I strongly felt that I should do more. I felt that I should use the energy that I had been shown, but I still had not worked out a system.

Depression is a terrible, disabling disease when it is not successfully treated. Because of how she felt, Maureen's adult daughter had driven her to our appointment. I was not sure of how I was going to help her but I thought to myself that I would trust and do my best.

When All Else Fails

Maureen and I sat down together in my clinic room, with her daughter present as well, as Maureen said she felt nervous. I felt for the familiar feeling that told me that Peter and Hiram were with me and then I began to speak, asking then why Maureen was so depressed. Maureen sat quietly in front of me.

"I see that you are struggling," I was told to tell her, *"It's because of the problem with her children,"*

"It is because of the problem with your children. You have not dealt with it."

"What problem?" she asked me when I repeated what I had been told to say.

I was told that Maureen had four children. I was puzzled as to why we were talking about children when she wanted to know about her depression. I was expecting hormonal imbalance, or celiac disease or something like that. Mentally I shrugged "You have four children?" I asked her.

"I have three children," she said, quite clearly Peter whispered to me and I sighed, sat back and listened some more. Then I opened my eyes and looked at her.

"You had better leave the room now," I told her daughter. The mother nodded to her and the daughter quietly got up and left.

"You have four children and your guilt is your depression."

Maureen began to cry. "I gave one away before we married. We couldn't keep him," She cried softly. Their children did not know that she and her husband had gone on to marry after putting their first baby up for adoption. Maureen's long held feelings of grief and guilt was still in her body, still in the way. She ached for the child she had relinquished and as a result, she was depressed and overweight. This was the first time that I was shown so clearly the connection between heart and body illnesses. I could see the depression in her body, in energy patterns. I could see it flowing in to all of her organs, her muscles, her bones, in short, her. The weight was protection from the sorrow and guilt.

But what did I do with this knowledge? How did I move this out of her?

Although I was not comfortable using Metatronic Energy on anybody else, I was shown myself using this energy on her in my mind. The compulsion to follow the 'instruction' was overwhelming so I asked Maureen to sit on a dining chair and then I stood behind her. I could feel my heart pounding with fear as Metatronic Energy dropped onto my hand. I could feel the coolness brushing across my palm and I knew that it was here. I also knew that it would not go into my body first, before being used on Maureen. The right hand pushes energy away and the left hand draws it in, therefore, calling Metatronic Energy onto your right hand means you can direct it and also keep it pure. This was what Metatron had instructed me to do when I was younger so I reasoned that it would be the same now.

I then dropped some Metatronic Energy into her, as I had been shown in the past and I directed this energy down through Maureen's body.

I was shown to ground her and I followed the instructions that I had been given when I used energy on myself. I asked Maureen to imagine herself plugged into the Earth through her base chakra, as my research had taught me that the base chakra was physically used to connect us to our family/traditional heritage and to the Earth. I then shielded her from negative emotions using gold as a protective frequency which was what my guides had shown me years before. Many people use white energy to seal them, but I had been shown that this was like using a spotlight on yourself.

I asked Maureen to do these exercises whenever she felt the need to and then we finished the session, with me feeling relieved that I had got through that experience.

But that was the beginning of using Metatronic Energy on other people. Maureen referred more people on to me and from that point on I would use this energy as part of every session. It would only take a few minutes to do this, and it always seemed to make people feel better. In fact, from the reports that I started getting back, it made a huge difference.

Maureen found her son.

The next problem, for me, was how to make this healing longer lasting. I wanted something that would make a difference and also stay more permanently in the body. I felt that a healing should last a few months if not forever, until a new issue was raised.

As I knew that the answer would be delivered to me when the time was right, I waited for the next piece of information to come to me. I had learned that there was no point in rushing it, or having a tantrum at my guides, though I still like to every now and then. It never made any difference. In the meantime I worked, and I got on with my life.

Finally, not long after I saw Maureen, I came home to a message written for me by my father. He had been looking after my sons, Harley and James and had answered the phone whilst I was out.

When I read the message I just about fell over with excitement. It was from Bernie.

I returned the call and Bernie answered. We talked for a while and he told me that he was now single. I told him that I was also single. We had not seen each other for years. I would have assumed that he had forgotten me but obviously he had not. We arranged to meet for dinner a few nights later and left it that. It would just be lovely to see him, I thought.

The night that we arranged to meet for dinner arrived. At 7.30pm there was a knock on the door and I walked down the hallway to open it. Bernie was standing on my verandah, looking through the wire door. He did not speak, but just stood there looking at me.

I opened the wire door up and stepped outside to join him, asking "Aren't you going to say hello?"

Bernie silently put his arms around me and hugged me. I was home.

We have been together every day since.

Chapter Fifteen:

Removing stories

March 1994

"Remove the story," a loud voice spoke clearly from somewhere behind me. Startled, I jumped and turned around, expecting to see someone, but I was alone, in my study at home.

I was not expecting to see or hear anyone, so I was a little disconcerted by the voice. It was just that I had not expected to hear someone – particularly a male someone – speak to me.

"Hello?" I asked, scanning the room. There was barely enough room for my desk, a bookshelf and two comfortable armchairs, let alone a lurking intruder, and I was fairly certain that it was a guide but it had seemed so loud, so separate that I thought I should be sensible and look. I walked out of the study and into the entry hall looking into the lounge-room. Empty. I moved back into the entry and opened the front door, glancing outside. No-one was in sight. I quickly walked around the rest of the house until I was satisfied that I was truly alone then I headed back to my study.

It was early in the day, my children were in daycare or at school and Bernie was at our clinic, working or getting stock for the small clinic to sell. We had married, happily, the year before.

I had taken the day off to be by myself, expecting to be by myself, not listening to disembodied voices again.

I sat down in one of the armchairs and mused for a while. Every now and then, out of the blue, Metatron would speak to me and give me a message. Sometimes I was lucky and I could understand the message, but sometimes it was as cryptic as 'remove the story'. I was not afraid of this voice, but I was perplexed. The messages were never very clear and often took a lot of sorting out. They were often just to be heard in my mind, but sometimes, like this message, they were out loud.

Now it was 'remove the story.'

I love books and I love stories. Perhaps it had meant for me to remove a book from my bookshelf and read it, waiting for the deeper meaning within to be revealed? The bookshelf in my study was full and even overflowing with novels of every description. I enjoy reading and I also enjoyed writing, and I was the editor of my own magazine –'*Spirit Eye*'. But what could this disembodied voice mean by telling me to 'remove the story'? What story? Which story? And remove it to where? How do I remove it?

I stared at the bookshelf for a while longer, allowing my eyes to scan over the list of books that I so enjoyed. Each and every tale within these books held meaning for me. I found deep truth in almost everything I read, picking the lessons of my life from within their pages. Often when I had a problem I would pick up a book, open it up and read what it said. It was funny how often what I read was relevant to my current situation.

I picked a book at random even though none of them were 'calling' me at this time, but it did not help. I put the book back into the shelf and sat down again.

I sat back in the comfortable armchair again, and closed my eyes, wanting to speak to one of my guides. I was an Aura Diagnostician/Medical Clairvoyant by profession and hearing disembodied voices was part of the job. Perhaps they could give me clarity.

What I doing now, as a Medical Clairvoyant, with the help of my guides, was to look at a person's energy system and ascertain where and why they had damaging blocks in the body and aura that was causing, or was about to cause, disease. Through trial and error I worked out that I could see which part of a body was unwell, whether that part was an organ, something in the blood or a gland. My internal mind would be directed to the area or areas. I had also worked out that there was an emotional cause, always, to each disease and I was able to intuit, what that emotional cause was. Just recently I had started to find familial links as well, so the whole thing seemed to have more depth and more clarity.

I really had fallen into this profession accidentally, or perhaps through being pushed by Spirit and I was the only person that I knew of who was doing this. People just seemed to find me, no matter where I went. There would be phone calls and someone had given them my number. I did not even have business cards.

I soon learnt that some talents that I had were unusual. I could see energy as it was discharged or created by the body. I could see the different colors that it was and the different shapes and patterns that it made. I could watch this energy as it changed when the person was upset, angry, drunk – anything. No-one else I knew of could do this, not even other healers that I had read about. I was also teaching clairvoyance and none of my students worked quite like me.

As I was inventing this profession of Medical Clairvoyance, I had no guidance and no help in the responsibilities or methods. There was no-one leading the way and there were no books explaining what I was seeing and what that could mean. Was this even real, or was I fooling myself? There was also no-one explaining to me how this could be useful or perhaps what moral guidelines I should follow.

I decided early in the piece that I should always be guided by both a moral sense and a good sense. I would do no harm and I would advise people that I am not medically trained and that they should always see a doctor to confirm my findings. I also realized that the more I was trained in anatomy and physiology and the more that I knew about medical procedures and drugs, the better I would be. So I set about learning as much as I could to be as knowledgeable as I could be. I was very lucky that Bernie went on to become an ambulance paramedic and he was able to guide me with things like medical procedures.

My energetic vision kept improving but the biggest problem for me was that I did not know what I could do about what I perceived in people. I could see if someone was developing lung cancer, for instance, but what good did this do for them, or me? Should I tell them about what I was seeing, or not? What if I saw something on a stranger in the street? And how should I tell them, and then what happened? When I spoke to anyone about my dismay over how I should handle this situation, I was often told that as least this person, my client, had a 'heads up', knowing that they were becoming ill months, or even years earlier than they would have known otherwise. I tried to content myself with this answer but it still was not enough.

By 1994 I had been a Medical Clairvoyant for about 10 years, but I wanted to be able to tell people what they could do to help themselves heal. The problem was all the available energy systems just seemed wrong to me and I had never heard of anyone else using Metatronic Energy. Nothing seemed to work in a deep and lasting sense. Everything seemed weak and hard to feel and when people tried to use them on me, they sort of washed away off me.

Each of them also felt wrong to me. In short, I had nothing recognized or formal, yet I knew that there was something waiting for me. If only I could find it. In the meantime here was I, doing something I had invented, using an energy that only I knew of. It was challenging.

I had my own clinic and I also had several medical doctors as clients. They had heard of me and were now clients themselves, quietly sending clients of theirs onto me, if needed. What I would do was discover a problem that was not yet gross enough to be easily found by standard tests.

Scientists had even travelled from as far away as England to study what I did, as had a scientist from Melbourne University, but none of this attention made me feel more useful or taught me what I could do to help people to heal more permanently.

I knew that I was looking for an energy that would clear the unwanted energy and rebuild the energy when I saw that it was weak or damaged. It seemed like Metatronic Energy should be able to do it, but I also knew that something was missing.

So I searched for something that would fit my wants. I was also trying to find something that would help people not call more illness to themselves so that these people could become truly well and empowered.

So far, it had been a long and fruitless search.

And now, out of the blue, one more time, came my friendly, disembodied voice –'Remove the story.'

I was puzzled but I let the mystery stand.

Less than a week after this event, my son James, who was four at this time, became ill but at first I did not know what was wrong; he just *looked* energetically sick to me. As I could see his energy I knew that *something* was wrong. Something critical seemed to be going on in his body and I was worried about him. Then he started to bruise a little. This didn't feel right and James didn't 'look' right. I could see that there was something odd with his immune system and something really wrong with his blood. He looked weak and sickly, energetically, to me. Physically he looked great but I made an appointment for him with our doctor and I asked her for a clotting factor test to be done because of the bruising.

Knowing me, she authorized the test I requested. I drove James from her clinic to the blood lab where blood was taken and a clotting test where they cut his arm and watched him bleed was performed. After a while the nurse called an end to the test and then James and I left for home.

As we walked in through the front door I could hear the phone ringing. By the time I had the door unlocked and open, with James running in front of me; Bernie was talking on the phone. I could hear Bernie speaking quietly then the phone was put down.

James ran into the family room to play and Bernie came up to me. "We need to go to the hospital," he said to me. I looked at him, puzzled. "That was Melbourne Pathology on the phone. You just had a test done on James?"

I nodded "Yes,"

"Well there's something wrong. We can't let him hit his head or hurt his stomach," Bernie went on explaining as we both heard the dull 'thud' of James' head cracking down on the tiled floor. I could feel my heart sink. "From this moment on, he can't hit his head," Bernie continued, unfazed. "He has almost no platelets."

I sighed. "Great," I said, walking to gather James up to go to the Royal Children's Hospital where he was to have more tests and the theory that they might remove his spleen was put to us.

It turned out that James had Idiopathic thrombocytopenic purpura (ITP). I did not care what he had. I was not letting them take his spleen without trying all other avenues. But what other avenues were there? We brought him home from hospital, determined to discover the problem that had caused the ITP myself.

I thought about his disease and how I was feeling. Frustrated. I couldn't prevent it, I couldn't say what it was and I couldn't heal it – I thought. But I thought that

I would try. And at least I had known something was wrong with him and where to start looking, that had given us a heads up in the race.

Then suddenly I knew what to do for James. I remembered Metatron's voice and his instruction to remove the story. I would remove the story, as I had been told to do.

My next question was how to do this. I felt quite unsure of how to proceed with the task but I also knew that I would be guided without too much fuss.

I went to find James and as I did I thought about his illness; the blood and not clotting and losing platelets. He was afraid to stick to anything and he had a lack of trust. His condition came from the heart chakra which rules emotions like love, acceptance of self and issues of commitment, to name a few. James held the stories within his body that were related to these issues. I knew that the way I had felt when I was pregnant with him had caused a lot of his illness now. These feelings had created the cells in his body and these cells related to the feelings of not being good enough, having to earn commitment, love, security. My heart felt like it was breaking for James.

His beginning to life had been fraught with peril. I had not been sure if he should be born at his time of birth. All the thoughts and all the fears that I experienced whilst pregnant with him must have had an impact, must have sat in his body, creating this disease. And indeed it did.

If I could remove the story, he would have fewer tantrums, he would be less fearful that I would abandon him and he would heal! No more blood tests and no more clotting problems.

If I could *not* remove the story, even if we healed the ITP, James would just develop something like Leukemia or Diabetes or any one of the other heart related conditions.

When I found James I had him sit on a stool, then I felt around for a feeling inside myself that felt right. If the Energy that I had always been shown felt wrong to me, then there *must* be one that feels right. I would look for that feeling. I closed my eyes and then I held out my hand.

In the short second that I was waiting for a response, I envisaged all sorts of scenarios in my mind. Flashes of me wearing flowing purple robes, or feathers on my head entered my brain. Dancing about chanting strange songs, banging gongs – all sorts of ridiculous scenarios kept flashing through my mind, and I was hard pressed to not burst in to laughter. I knew that I could not ever do this and if that is what it took, I was afraid I was not going to be able to help.

In my mind I called to this Voice that had been speaking to me, to show me what I needed. Immediately I could feel a quiet laughter in response to my imaginings and all the ridiculous images faded. 'Keep it simple…' came the instruction. I admit that I was relieved.

After a few minutes I could feel something on my hand, on my right hand. When I was sure that I could feel the Energy – it was a cool tingling pressure – I dropped this Energy into James' Crown Chakra and then I began to direct it as I had been told to do. I could feel this Energy as it moved down his body, and more importantly, James could feel it too. I trusted that I would be further guided. I was 'impressed' to move my hands slowly down his body, stopping briefly over each major Chakra point until I could feel the Energy on each of my hands, back and front of his body.

After a few minutes I stopped running the Energy and then all we could do was wait. There felt like something more that I should do, or show James to do, but I did not know what it could be. I resolved to keep exploring until I found it, then I gave James a hug and sent him off to play. I knew that the next lesson would come to me. All I had to do was be patient.

I used this new Energy on James a few times each week, and James was looking healthier and healthier after each time. Although he started having major tantrums again and I was not sure of why that was but obviously something was shifting in him. James had had a few really big tantrums in his life, particularly if he thought I was leaving him, and also when a young cousin of his had died very suddenly. These events had thrown James of target and now he was having similar symptoms again.

As he and I worked together, with Energy as our tool, we talked about what he could feel and what dreams he was having at nights. His dreams told me that we were doing the right thing and that he was getting better. I just wanted to make the tantrums go away.

Every week or so James and I would go back to the children's hospital for more tests, but James became more and more stressed with each visit. Finally, the test results were almost normal and I refused to allow them to continue. He was meant to have this condition for a long time. He was meant to be tested until they were convinced that it was not leukemia or something else lurking, but I judged that we had this condition under control.

About three months later I organized another test. James' blood test results were now normal. He had recovered from this condition in record time, without complications. But the tantrums continued until I was given the next part of the puzzle.

That was more than 15 years ago. James is 19 years old now at the time of writing this book, 195cms tall and healthy. He has just discovered the delights of cooking for himself and I still run energy through him when he is sick, at his request.

Sometimes he goes to a doctor.

November 1994

'Remove the story and throw them away…' I am sure I heard that.

Throw them away? It was the same feeling that I had had before, a disembodied voice with a cryptic message. It had been about 6 months since I had heard the voice last and the message seemed now to have changed. Was this the information I had been waiting for?

I was sure that it was Metatron, who was talking to me. Hiram came to me whenever I called, as did my other Guides, Peter, and now Rondor and Alexander.

But so far they had not enlightened me, even when questioned. They just seemed to shrug and wander off. Was it a secret? Obviously it was, but why? It seemed that it was only Metatron who could tell me what to do with this, but that I had to get good at dealing with one part before he gave me another part.

So far I had the energy he had given, I was told to remove the story, to keep the procedure simple. He had shown me how to do that in such a way that it only took a few minutes for human intervention and then the energy itself would do the rest. I was told to use my right hand to call the energy, the left hand to draw it through the body. So few and surprisingly simple instructions for such a strong energy and now the next one was to throw it away.

My new instruction: 'throw them away'. That made sense.

I had a new problem now that I was dealing with and again it was with James and his tantrums. As I had used this Energy his tantrums had become worse, and it became even more obvious than ever that he had a 'problem'. I was sure that James was an Asperger. He had all the symptoms; the disconnectedness, the inability to understand other people's emotions, the obsession with systems, and in James' case – trains.

James' tantrums had continued on since I had begun using Metatronic Energy on him. They had eased off a lot and were almost gone, but they were still a focus that I wanted gone.

I am a very mild Asperger and I had been raised in a family with more than one around me so I was in no rush to have my child diagnosed and boxed. There was no real help for anyone in the spectrum and these Aspergers seemed to be mostly met with aggression and derision. If given a choice between knowledge and ignorance, I was certainly wishing I could be ignorant.

In James' short life he had had the ITP: he had also been suspected of having a brain tumor and Epilepsy when he was about 18 months old, but fortunately both conditions had turned out to be negative. But by now I was emotionally tired and he was not yet four years old.

I wanted James to go to a normal school, with other normal people and I was determined that this bright, energetic and determined boy would do just that. I wanted him to learn how to make friends. So far, when he saw a child that he liked he would rush up to them and make faces at them, then rush away just as suddenly. So far, he had not had much success with his technique.

I put the problem of James aside and sat back in the chair in my study and began to meditate on the problem of this disembodied voice speaking to me *again*. First of all, who was it that was speaking to me? And why were they speaking to me? Now we were up to *'throw them away…'*

I asked my guides to show me who this being really was. I had no idea – none at all. I let my mind drift, thinking about stories, my life, where I wanted to be, where I was now. Wondering how I had come such a long way away from the life I thought I would have, to this life…

Carmel Bell

Remembering Metatron

'It is Metatron.' came the voice inside my mind.

'Hiram,' I responded, 'Hello.' The sensation of a smile, warmth floods my body. I sense Hiram, tall, browned, Egyptian and bald. My friend, my husband in many lives, a doctor in his last life and now again, a doctor for me, in this my lifetime.

'Hello,' came the reply. 'It is Metatron.' He said again, simply and quietly.

Okay – Metatron it is. 'Throw them away?' I asked 'Throw what away? The story?' I asked.

Hiram laughed. I could feel the warmth inside me. 'Yes. The story that you all carry, all souls carry their stories. These are the stories that make you sick. You keep holding onto them. You move them through but then cling to them as if they were precious pieces of gold. Throw them away.' I could see images of people arguing, me arguing, moments of pain, moments of disappointment or anguish. Hurts from all my life flooded past me in a rush. I think I was starting to understand. The stories…stories from our childhoods, patterns that formed from the first moment we drew breath, stories that were handed to us from our families, expectations, fears, good times and bad. Stories that make us expect some things and be afraid of others. These stories lurked in the cells of our bodies and created disease and disharmony. And then it was the same story, over and over and over, again and again. The same lover, the same friend, even if it was a different person, a different body. We found the same story because that is what we are used to. My head filled up with all the images and all the information. How simple it really was, to be done with a situation, truly done, and not keep reliving it. We are a transmitter and we will find what we call to, until we change the signal. We change the signal by finding the story, then throwing it away. This is what I had been missing. I could not afford to cling onto these stories any longer. None of us could.

If we could find the story and remove it, it was like pulling a toxin out of a body and then administering an antidote. I had been finding the story, but I had not been throwing the story away. No wonder James had been getting worse.

"Show me how." I asked.

'You use the energy you have been given…' I could see a rubbish bin in my mind and I was tempted to laugh.

Hiram faded and I could feel a tingling, quite clearly on my hand and on my crown chakra - a warm, crisp tingle that kept on running, without fading. I could feel this energy as it moved down through my crown and into my body. It felt right. This was the energy that I used on James, myself and my clients, but I had never felt Metatronic Energy as strongly or as clearly as this before then. It I was excited. I knew that I had gone up a level in my ability.

'Hiram! It's great!'

I knew that this new level was able to shift the stories out of the body and to discard them so that you would be truly free of them.

This was the answer that I had been waiting for. I now felt like I had most of the puzzle at my fingertips. I knew how to read the energy system and the chakras and in the last few months I had worked out how to call energy to ferret out the stories from the body, altering the energy within us. Now I had been shown how to find that energy without searching and more importantly, how to discard the stories. I could finally and completely get rid of the story. I was excited.

As I continued to sit quietly in my study, my memory was suddenly flooded with memories of Metatron and more answers were given to me. I knew the answer. Metatron was an Archangel – the Archangel. He was the right hand of God and was the bridge between Heaven and Earth. Metatron means between worlds or the 'Great Transformation' and legend has it that if you want to speak to God, you spoke to Metatron.

I was shown Metatron kneeling down to talk to me when I was four – the same age as James was now. Suddenly his message flooded back into me. The knowledge of how I was to use energy to see what was wrong with people. How I was to use Energy to remove the toxins from their bodies, how I was, in short, to be a Medical Intuitive. All this came flooding back in a flash.

Now, apparently, he wanted to speak to me again.

I first met Metatron when I was four years old. I died briefly and whilst having a Near Death Experience, I was introduced to Metatron. He asked me to pass his energy on, but as I grew up, the experience faded. I forgot about what he had asked me to do, but all through my life, I had been guided by him. I recognized now the voice as his. He was the voice in the dark, the voice that warned me of danger, or asked me to change direction. Now he was talking to me in my study, apparently to have me remove the story.

The 'Voice' laughed at my memories. 'Yes,' he spoke, 'You are to remove the stories. That is how you will heal people.' Inside my mind I could see the same images of people arguing and I could see the cells that made the body being altered by all this distress. Then I was shown the cells being changed as the process was reversed, the stories removed. With each letting go, more toxins would flee the body and the cells would rejuvenate. With each letting go, recreation would be possible.

I was shown James and how we had healed him by using this energy but because I did not remove the story that had made him sick, it had risen up and initiated tantrums. I could have avoided these tantrums if I had listened earlier. Some of James' tantrums would last for hours. He was legendary. (He is incredibly peaceful now.)

Ahhh! So that's how it is done. I remove the story from the cell. The stories create the cells! And then we discard the story. So simple.

Then something more occurred to me. James, my son, I had been rattling the stories through him and although all of him was getting healthier, it seemed that the Asperger part was becoming more pronounced. Could I use any of this that I had learnt to help James?

I asked Metatron and he showed me that because we were altering James to improve his life, his Asperger way was becoming highlighted. Eventually, it would be more dominant.

'Can I stop this?' I asked. Aspergers are brilliant people. If we could keep the brilliance but give him normalcy, I would be overwhelmed. This would prove to me that what I was being taught was worth passing on.

Metatron laughed quietly and warmly. I was shown an image of James learning to imitate people, practicing the skills that he needed so that he could fit in. What he was showing me was choosing to be different, choosing to replace a dysfunction with something better. 'Any ideas as to how I can do this for James?' Into my mind came the image of Thomas the Tank Engine. I was a little puzzled and was about to ask more. But before I could there was a knock on my study door.

The door opened and Bernie poked his head in. "Hello," he smiled at me. "I got you something." He held out a book to me.

"Hello," I smiled at Bernie as I stood up to kiss him. I held out my hand and took the book, kissing him at the same time. I stepped back slightly and looked at the book he had given me – '*Anatomy of Spirit* by Caroline Myss'. Finally I had found someone who did something like me.

James learned to be like other people through the use of this energy and the watching of Thomas the Tank Engine videos. He also taught himself to read through these videos. He did so well that he appears normal now.

The importance of knowledge

Life got into a pattern. I went to work, I looked after my children and I used the knowledge that I had been given. I would see a client, diagnose what was wrong, run energy into them, and teach them how to handle this energy and how to remove the stories from their bodies. Then we would talk about how they could replace this old story with something better.

I was also doing a lot of pro-bono work, which took up a lot of time. Bernie and I had two more children together but both of our children had been born prematurely and quite unwell and I also had a stroke during the birth of our daughter, our youngest child. Because I used Metatronic Energy to heal myself, I healed rapidly and almost completely. Really only Bernie and I could tell.

I used Metatronic Energy on myself to turn the damage around and I also used it to heal our children whilst they were in hospital. Our youngest son also had two strokes, one at day four and one at day ten, but he is fine now. He is completely normal and on par with his peers.

Bernie and I were both very busy. My practice always remained consistent, but it always felt like something was still lacking. I wanted the *'great story'* to tell, the something that convinced me that this really worked. I had enough people who were prepared to state that I helped, but I was not convinced.

In about 1999 I started to notice that there was something wrong with me. I just did not feel right and when I scanned my body I could see a shadow on my brain, around the site of the pituitary gland.

Our daughter was about one year old at this stage. I started travelling more for work, going to the UK and to America to teach Medical Intuition and Metatronic energy. There seemed to be a quiet groundswell happening with this energy that I had been given, but I still did not feel as if I had enough evidence that I could talk about it with authority.

My clinic got busier and busier, my courses more booked out and I was getting sicker and sicker, even though on the outside, I looked fine. I could feel it and see it in my energy system. I also knew that I was feeling frustrated with my practice. I wanted to help people and I felt that to do so, I needed something that could convince people that this energy had something to offer and was not just energy.

Meditating one day about what to do to help reach more people with this energy, I spoke to my guides and I asked them why I was feeling so tired. 'Cushings Disease.' came the whispered response. I immediately went and did some research on Cushings. What I discovered was that Cushings was caused by a tumor on the pituitary gland. I looked at photos of people who had Cushings and they were all huge, with fat bodies and skinny arms and legs. The tales that they told of their life and their treatment was terrible.

I took myself to the doctor and asked for a referral to an endocrinologist. Then I made an appointment. I was very lucky that I have this ability to read energy and that I have doctors who will trust me and help me. Because I saw the tumor on my pituitary gland Cushings disease was diagnosed in me years before it would have otherwise been. I was also able to avoid a lot of the devastation that goes hand in hand with Cushings.

I used Metatronic Energy to keep myself going for 10 years without treatment. I could never manage to rid myself of the tumor which was a major disappointment, but I kept it under control.

I started my college in February 2008 and in also in 2008 I decided to have the tumor removed. I knew that the chances of success, at least the first time, were slim, but I was tired and I was willing to take the chance.

I had the tumor removed in December 2008, with the plan of being back at work in February. I don't know what I was looking forward to more; looking normal again as I had put on about 10 kilos and my face had got round, or having a non work related break.

The surgery went smoothly, with no complications and I looked forward to life becoming more normal again.

Even though I was deeply disappointed that I had had to have the surgery, I was prepared to accept it and move on with life. The best laid plans and all that.

Carmel Bell

Thinking about life

January 2009: Post surgery. I thought back on my life again, to the time that we first had it confirmed that my son James was an Asperger, to where he is now, almost completely normal. I also thought about my other children and how the two youngest had both been premature and not expected to live and how I had used Metatronic Energy to save them and to make them healthy. It has been a remarkable energy to me. I have been blessed beyond belief.

By 2009 I had spent 15 years teaching this energy – Metatronic Energy – to people. I was also working in my clinic, working five days a week and I was also running a college that I had opened to teach Medical Intuition.

But I still felt lost and unfulfilled. I still felt as if I did not have the evidence I needed to show people that it truly was simple, that they could heal their body and their heart and live a fulfilled life. I still felt as if the last piece of the puzzle was missing.

I remembered back to being handed the book by Caroline Myss and being so excited to have been given this book and then to read it. Her book explained so much of what I was doing, and gave it a title, but it was not all of what I was doing. I was also disappointed because she was so different to me.

We were different and I wanted to be able to explain how we different. I was more traditionally medical and I also liked to heal people and empower them.

When All Else Fails

The differences were not huge but they were remarkable. My problem was that I needed to convince myself.

I did not feel that I had what I needed, not yet, not until I died. I had a lot of clients who could attest that I have helped them but I wanted something more. I wanted the dead person walking.

I kept on feeling lost and I kept on waiting for the story that was incredible enough for me to use to show people how energy could actually work.

Then February 15th, 2009 I was given the story that I needed for me to talk about.

In my sleep, *for no known reason*, I suffered from a sudden cardiac arrest and was dead for 47 minutes, medically recorded time. During those 47 minutes I received CPR, seven electric shocks and s six shots of adrenaline.

But more importantly in that time I was able to talk to Metatron, face to face. He told me himself what it was he wanted, and needed me to do. It was through his grace and his energy that I am able to be here today, writing this book so that you can read about his energy, without me having brain damage, despite my medically recorded, medically proven, completely unarguable time spent dead, and then return to life *with brain damage*. It took me 10 months to restore my brain function to this point, from having a five minute memory, to being able to remember most of my life again, from not being able to recognize my home to being able to drive again and from not being able to stand upright, to being able to run and to being normal.

Here I am. This is his energy.

Chapter Sixteen:

Waking up dead

I'm dead. I thought as I woke up. Feeling surprised, I looked at the clock.

The bedside clock on the other side of the room glowed 3.09 AM. It was Sunday, February 15, 2009.

I'm dead, I thought again, involuntarily, as I looked down at my body lying in bed: I could see my physical body quite clearly. *My body?* Shocked, surprised and slightly horrified, I looked again.

I'll be damned! I think I am dead! I was astounded and I could feel the first tendrils of panic curling around inside of me and I really did not want to panic. I swallowed the feeling and began to think. How did I get here, to being dead? How was I going to recover?

I tried lying back down inside my body. I sat on myself and tried settling back into me, and just as quickly found myself back on the edge of the bed, sitting next to myself and I knew that, no matter what I did I would not be allowed 'back in'.

Yep. Definitely dead. I sighed and began to think. What had I done?

I'd gone to bed tired but happy after attending my cousin's wedding. I had drunk a glass of champagne during the wedding festivities and I had also danced, but I did not think that this would have killed me.

I'm dead, I thought again as I looked at my body lying in bed: I could see my physical body quite clearly. Knowing that I was out of my body was in itself not worrying, but realising that I was dead was, particularly as I was clearly not going to be allowed back in easily. I wasn't quite sure how I got out of my body and I was not sure how I was going to get back in but I knew that there had to be a way. Just to check, I tried lying down on myself again but that did not work. I found myself sitting up next to my body again.

I realized that I was out of my body, not because I chose to be but because I had been 'kicked out' of it. My body and my consciousness were separate from each other. This was dead and I was no longer welcome inside my 'home'. *That's a weird thought*, I thought to myself.

I did not feel panic. Not yet. I noted that I could also not feel any pain. And I definitely had no idea what had killed me. Slowly, I looked over my body as if this was a problem I could solve. I scanned 'me' to see if I could see any blood or anything else that was obvious. Perhaps I would see a knife sticking out of my chest, or some expression of horror on my face. I was looking for anything that would give me a clue so that I would know what to do. But my eyes were closed and I looked peaceful.

I was aware that "I", my consciousness, was sitting on the bed. I had a body but the body felt different. For starters, we felt separate from each other. I, what I was now, felt real, but my body was not weighty or solid. I was also surprised at how well I could see inside my bedroom, considering that it was night-time.

Bernie, my husband, was sleeping, lying undisturbed next to my body, and the bedside clock was now showing 3.11am.

Two minutes.

Two minutes since I had first noticed the time.

With a dull sense of shock I realized again that I was dead. I wanted back in, but not because I was so attached to my body that I couldn't go on without it. Then I realized something. *'I can't live without it!'* I reeled in shock, but also noticing how, even without the physical body, I could still feel my head spinning.

I sat on the edge of the bed next to myself and began to think hard. Now, when I thought about it I realized I was not really surprised at this sudden event, as for months my guides had been telling me that I was going to die, that my heart was going to fail. It seemed that each time I turned on the radio, the song "This heart attack" by the band, Faker, had been playing, but I could never find anything wrong with my heart no matter how many times I had 'scanned' it.

Even so, I was still surprised by this turn of events. Why now? Why tonight? I'd gone to bed healthy and feeling well. The last thing I expected was to wake up literally dead. I was swinging between saying to myself "What?!" to "Oh well," and accepting the outcome.

But to find myself literally sitting and looking at my own body was disturbing. What was I supposed to do? How was I to behave? There were no protocols for suddenly finding yourself dead. No self help book on the topic -'Waking up Dead! What to do when all else is done!' But...

Dead? Yes, I was sure of that. I wasn't breathing. This wasn't a dream, nor was it a normal out-of-body experience. This was death. How could I tell? I could tell because this felt different. I felt disconnected from me and when I tried to re-enter me, I could not.

I sat quietly thinking about things for a few moments. What should I do? What did I want to do? I honestly had no idea, then I looked at Bernie, lying unaware next to my body and I knew. I wanted to live with him. Bernie and I are strongly connected. People would call us 'soul mates'. We are happiest when we are together and I could not imagine being dead and being without him.

I looked around my bedroom and it looked the same. There was no light, no tunnel appearing. I was happy about that, but also a touch uneasy. What if 'The Light' never appeared? What if I was stuck here forever? I could not imagine many worse things than being a ghost. Panic rose in my throat and I swallowed it again, quickly. I had died briefly when I was four and the light and the tunnel had appeared then, so I was reasonably confident that it would appear again, eventually.

I willed myself back to calm and surprisingly, I was able to succeed. Then, still sitting, I once more looked at the clock. It was now 3.15 AM. How long had I been dead? I was not sure but it had been six minutes since I had first noticed the time on the clock. So I had been dead for at least six minutes.

With each second that passed, I knew that since I wasn't breathing and my cells weren't receiving oxygen, more cells were dying in my body. My brain cells were flickering out, like a rolling blackout striking the lights of a vast night-time city, and my Energy system looked dull.

Oxygen, I thought, *I need oxygen.* I willed my body to breathe. I tried to grab my physical shoulder, so that I could shake my body, but I was just an energy form and this had no effect. My body remained totally still on the bed. I thumped my chest and my hand just passed through, no feeling in my hand at all. There was absolutely no connection, and in such a way that I had never felt before in this lifetime, not even when I had briefly died before.

My spirit had left my body: the object lying in the bed beside my sleeping husband was clay. I knew I was dead. I knew that this was different to the astral travelling kind of experience or my previous NDE because I felt no attachment to my body, at all. Someone could have hacked my body apart with a chainsaw and I would have felt nothing.

Even when you astral travel, you still maintain awareness, a connection to your body. If someone was to tickle you, or stab you, you would feel it still through your connection. Just as people who have been hurt whilst they were out of their body or under anaesthetic have known that something has happened to them, even if they were not aware of all of the details.

Now my body was Earth. *Earth to Earth*, I thought. But I wasn't prepared to die. I had too much I wanted to do and see.

Once more emotion reared up in me. I could feel it, thick in my throat with its presence, a fierce determination to not give in, to not be told what I was going to do.

Damn! I thought. I knew I needed help, fast. But how could I get help?

On the other side of the bed, completely oblivious to my situation, Bernie slumbered on. I felt a flash of sadness for him. I knew he would never recover from my death. I can only imagine how awful that would be, to wake in the morning next to someone you loved, to find them dead. All the expectations that we had created of a life together, like a future, laughter, fun, travel, love – all gone. All the things we put off today because we are certain that we will have a tomorrow. All ripped away. I could not imagine how that would feel, to lose that simple trust.

Wake up, Bernie, I thought. *Please wake up.*

3.16AM. Seven minutes gone. More brain cells dead. My body needed oxygen. I knew that unless I got help quickly, my condition would be permanent; I'd never wake up again. *How long can my brain survive without oxygen before I am beyond help?* I wondered.

Now I was definitely starting to feel apprehensive. My body lay on its back, my left arm flung up and covering my face. A person can survive less than five minutes without oxygen. Without oxygen, the human brain starts to die. And I knew I had already gone beyond the five minute mark.

My husband is a paramedic, an ambulance officer. I needed his skills. He had to try to resuscitate me, and quickly. But he was asleep. I felt a moment of resignation because, even if I was resuscitated now I knew that I would have brain damage already. I wondered how that would appear. Would I lose intelligence, memory, or social graces? Would I be in a wheelchair, drooling?

Would I become aggressive? All of these scenarios would be possible and none of them are desirable. I very nearly quit right then. I would much rather be dead than burdening my family with a liability.

Everything is energy, I reminded myself. If it is broken, surely it can be fixed. For now, all I had to do was focus my energy and jolt him awake, so that he could see what was happening.

I calmed myself down and then I pulled as much of my energy into me as I could. "Wake up, Bernie!" I shouted, not knowing if he could hear me or not, but I had to try. "Wake up – can't you see that I'm dead?" I shoved my energy at him, pushing him energetically, but he slumbered on.

3.17AM. the bedside clock ticked away another minute. Eight minutes gone.

Desperately I focused all my energy on Bernie: I had to get him to wake up. "Bernie! Help me!" I concentrated as hard as I could and kept concentrating. I was also dimly aware of something else in my consciousness... I was aware of Heaven...? That was all I could think it could be, but I ignored it. I had to wake Bernie up and I could not afford to be distracted.

3.18AM. Bernie moved and turned over.

"Help me. I need you now; I need you to wake up, please Bernie."

I was surprised at how long I had been dead for, without 'Heaven' appearing and sweeping me off. *How much longer do I have?* I wondered as I fought to contain the desperation I could feel growing in my chest.

Nine minutes had passed. To my relief, Bernie sat up. "Look at me," Bernie, I directed him. "Please look at me now."

Yawning, Bernie stood up and blundered out of the bedroom.

I could only watch in disbelief. I was dead and my husband was going to the bathroom! *I'll laugh about this one day*, I thought as I sat back to wait for Bernie's return.

Although death is a continuation of life, when you stop breathing, the billions of cells of the human body stay alive, some of them for hours, but inevitably, the longer that there's no life-giving oxygen, the more of your cells die: in your blood, in your organs, and in your brain.

3.19AM. Ten minutes dead.

Bernie came back. "Look at me, Bernie. Look at me," I ordered him with all the force I could. "Please help me. It's almost too late."

Bernie lay down beside me again. He looked so sweet, half asleep. He lay on his side, facing me and put his arm around me, cuddling me.

I can't do it, I thought. *I can't wake him. He'll wake hours from now and I'll be dead*. I lay down on the bed, in between Bernie and my body, up close to him. I could not feel his warmth. I wanted to cry, but I whispered to him, right in his ear, *'I'm sorry.'*

Bernie sat up and switched on the lamp. I could feel his confusion, he knew that something was wrong, but he didn't know what it was.

3. 20 Am. Eleven minutes dead.

He looked at my body and said my name. "Carmel…"

Bernie removed my hand from my face and shook me. He stared at me. He knew what a lifeless body looked like. "What have you done!?" Bernie asked me in a kind of quiet shout. I could hear and feel the desperation, the shock in his voice. I could also feel how his body was vibrating slightly and I knew that adrenaline must be coursing through him

Yelling to our son, James, he jumped out of bed, switching on the main bedroom light. Bernie left the room and I waited next to my body. I started to relax now and feel safe. I also had more time to observe how I was feeling and how I was reacting. It was as if time was doing weird leaps, jumping from one scene to another. It was more fluid than normal time but also less solid. Thought had a profound effect on what I saw and what I felt. I could slow time down, or speed it up, by willing it.

Whilst I was watching time/space behaving differently, I was also aware that I could hear Bernie talking. I realized that I could see, feel and *be* in more than one place at a time.

Suddenly he was back in our room. He climbed onto the bed and knelt over my body. Bernie started CPR. I could absently 'feel' the pressure on my chest, the air being forced into my lungs, but it was as if I had been numbed. It felt like I had been given a local anaesthetic all over, but it was an odd kind of feeling. It was real, but not quite real. I felt still attached to my body, but no longer in it, or of it, but the caretaker of it. There was no pain.

Bernie knew what he was doing. He is an incredibly capable man and I knew that if anyone could help me, it would be him. But I had been dead for at least eleven minutes.

My dead body's breathing would start again very soon, I hoped. The rest of it was now up to me.

Chapter Seventeen:

Heaven

Death ... is no more than passing from one room into another.
- Helen Keller

When you are dead, you are still a 'consciousness', but your 'consciousness' feels global as well as local. You have a body, but the body is made up of energy instead of flesh. The energy body *appears* as if it is flesh but it is a different density and frequency to the spiritual body. The spiritual body does have limits because you have limits in your consciousness. The physical body has limits because it has physical boundaries. You cannot out learn your brain; you cannot outrun your legs. You can improve them, but they are still finite, dependant on your IQ, your genetics, your flexibility and more.

In spirit because you have no limit on the size or capacity of your brain, anything is possible, depending on your consciousness or recognition of the possibility. If you want to walk, you will walk but if you want to fly, then you will soar.

And with a 'spiritual' brain you can learn several things at once; you can also hold knowledge of several lifetimes or timelines with ease. The human brain is like a single drawer filing cabinet whereas the spiritual brain is like an entire library of filing cabinets. In spirit, you can be aware of many things at once; it all depends on where you focus your attention. Now my attention turned from what was happening with my physical body, to something else that I'd been aware of since I woke up out of my body -there was a feeling in me as if there was someone watching me; someone that I could not see, yet knew was there. I stood still and relaxed.

Suddenly, Heaven was here. I realized that Heaven was all around me and had been all around me all along. There was no transition from Earth to Heaven but there was a visual shimmering of the air and then there I was aware of a different sensation and a different feel. I was in heaven.

At the age of four, when I'd had a near death experience (NDE), I had experienced the classic scenario of going through the tunnel and to the light – all the accoutrements of an NDE. From being dead this time I know that if you experience a classic NDE, you are actually *not* meant to be dead, you are meant to live. You will go back to your body. Going down the 'tunnel' into the light is like going into the waiting lounge at an airport. You are in transit and not meant to stay in Heaven. I had had similar experiences when I had died on the operating table at 17 and also after my son, James, was born in 1991.

This time, my fourth NDE experience, was different. When I first realized that I was both conscious and also dead, I kept waiting for the light and the tunnel to appear. It didn't feel strange at the time to realize that I was both alive and dead but I was relieved that the light and the tunnel did not appear, even though my vaguely formed plan had been to run around the room, keeping out of the way if it did appear.

But now that Bernie had discovered my body, I was ready to leave. I knew that if I did not go to 'Heaven' then I would stand *no* chance of coming back. I looked around my room and even though there was still no light or tunnel, I became part of heaven more easily than going from one room to another. It was as simple as deciding that I was ready to be there.

As soon as I let myself relax enough to shift awareness I was finally in Heaven. I realized that I had already been there. I was already there. Straightaway I started to look around me.

The first thing that emotionally registered was a disappointment that there was no one there to greet me. I assumed all my life that when I died there would be people there to collect me. That I was on my own, physically, was an emotional blow. There was nobody there to greet me or to help me. I was standing alone.

I decided to look around me and take stock of my surroundings.

Stars were in the dark sky above me and flickers of energy shone all around me, but these flickers were not right at my face level or in the air right in front of me where I might touch them. They were several feet away from me, above me. These energies were literally stunning –I think that the closest thing I could humanly align them to would be the Australian Aboriginal min min lights.

It also felt like I was standing on the edge of the world, slightly above Earth, looking down, but there was no edge or cliff to walk up to. This was just how it felt – as if there was no end and yet there was definitely an end. As strange as it may sound to say, because I did not have a physical body, I was also aware of myself physically. I noticed that I was not aware of feeling heat or cold, yet I could still feel emotion. I felt a huge, unsettled mixture of feelings, from awe, to being saddened by being dead so suddenly and so unexpectedly. I was also feeling alone. My expectations were that when you 'arrive' in Heaven, there would be some sort of welcoming party to greet you as this was what I had read, again and again.

Maybe these beings would explain how it works, where you should go, show you where you can rest and generally answer questions for you. After all, even though you had been dead before, it may have been quite some time ago, or even a shock to your system, if, like me, you were not truly expecting to die.

Every story I had ever read about NDE's talked about the people or beings they had met. Putting my expectations aside, knowing that I had no time to be concerned about it now, I continued with my self appraisal. Although I knew I didn't have the physical body I was used to, I discovered that I was still the energy which is me, and my non-physical energy body could move, think and speak. I knew that it could not suffer injury or illness, but it could suffer heartache. I was not suddenly wiser, smarter, and I assume no prettier, because I was already everything that I had become.

My recognition of this meant that everything in my universe was the same and yet completely different. I became keenly aware that on Earth I was *already* the composite of all my previous life experiences. I had carried forward with me all the lessons that I had learned in previous lives and I was at the level of spiritual development that I was at because I have lived a thousand lives before this one. Just because I could not say "Oh yes, when I was Alexander the Great's primary physician, I learnt how to reattach a finger that had been amputated back onto a hand." did not mean that I did not have that knowledge somewhere inside of me.

To become a healer like a Medical Intuitive, you need to be an experienced soul. Although it is largely unseen, the energy that I use and teach for my profession is powerful and effective and it is not placed into the hands of an unwise soul. If you are called to a healing profession such as this, it is a large soul responsibility.

As I continued my observation I became very aware that although I was in Heaven, yet I was also still attached to my room. This small piece of seemingly unimportant knowledge has changed me and my life almost more than anything else. Heaven is right here. Right where you are, right now, so is Heaven.

I realized that Heaven and my room were the same space in the Universe, even though they were different dimensions to each other, which is how they, Heaven and Earth, *can and do* occupy the same place. Every place on earth and in the Universe is in Heaven. This knowledge explained so much to me, about how spirit guides could be real and could send information to people on earth. They step from their dimension into ours. As they can go back and forth through time, they can tell you how your future is going to turn out. The real trick is learning how to listen to these beings clearly, without your own interpretation.

I was also given information on how space travel and other alien species that we will eventually meet. I was excited to have this knowledge drop straight into my brain.

Whilst thinking about all this I was also aware of other thoughts in my brain. I noticed that my attention, my brain capacity, could be focussed on several things at once, which is how people who undergo an NDE can come back with phenomenal tracts of information. Time is not necessary to learning when you are in spirit. It is more a question of what you want to know.

As I scanned my body I wished that I had a mirror because I could not see my face. I would have liked to know for sure that I still looked like me.

Even so, I could see my chest, arms, legs, and clothing that I was wearing. My body looked and felt exactly as I should, but I felt no discomfort, or pressure, or physical awareness of anything touching me. To have none of these physical boundaries is actually a little weird and disconcerting. It is very like floating in space, without clothes on.

Although I knew that I was standing, I could not 'feel' the place beneath my feet, yet I knew that it was there. There was an awareness of ground, without their being any sense of pressure on my feet. I was also not floating and I was not falling. I was standing, as I expected to be, and there were no beings floating or flying around me anywhere either. I knew that it was only a matter of time before I adjusted to this way of being, of being physically aware without the need for physical discomfort. It was pretty much the same as being on

Earth with the ground, the sky above and an upright position in the world.

When I concentrated on the ground, sometimes it seemed like it was grass and other times it seemed like it was just nondescript ground.

The longer that I stood there, the more *real*, the more *solid* Heaven became to me and the more that my awareness of my body and what it/I was experiencing in my bedroom, decreased. I knew that this shift in awareness was happening very rapidly. This must be the process that we all go through when we die with the gradual letting go of the body.

And I realized again, far more strongly, that Heaven is here, right here. Heaven was with me all along and always has been here. Heaven is where we are, wherever we are, whatever planet we are on. Whether we are in an aeroplane, on a yacht, or climbing a mountain or travelling to distant planets, Heaven is right with us. It is not an up or a down place, but it is a place that is wherever we are. It never leaves you and spirit really does here you when you cry for help. I wonder why, even now, the answer is sometimes 'No' when we desperately want a 'Yes'. And then the knowledge that sometimes what we think we want or need would be the worst thing for us was given to me. I accept this, but I still argue it.

Nevertheless, once I had realized that heaven was here, Heaven opened to me. It had never left me, not since the moment I had first reincarnated. I have always been in Heaven. I just could not see it.

I also realized that although we are Spirit, and prescribed a higher purpose, I knew that I could run, walk, laugh and dance, should I so choose to. I could do those things that we might consider to be silly and Human and 'beneath' us. I knew that if I chose to, I could live a full life, with the other people who were here in heaven. It would be a different life to the one that I had been living. Information is rapidly gained once in spirit. There is no need to absorb by reading or other methods. Knowledge of how the Universe runs is just there. I think this knowledge is why some people seem to be born with a natural understanding of how things *could* be, or *should* be as opposed to how they currently are. I think this is how the great minds, like Leonardo Da Vinci was so inventive, from remembering all the things he had known about in Heaven.

Because of this I also knew that I could visit, or see, Earth as well as other planets if I wanted to, but what I could not do was feel the pleasures of the flesh. We neither eat nor have sex in Heaven and I know that this is why so many people have problems with both those activities. They are overwhelmed by the abundant feelings that these activities rouse in them when they feel them.

I started to wonder to myself why it was that I could still be so *alive* when my body was so clearly dead. Was it because I was still attached to my body, or because I was undergoing CPR? Did that keep me connected or was there some other answer? Was it just that the flesh was dying, but the essential 'me', the Carmel, was alive regardless? Would I go onto my next life with Carmel essentially a part of me still?

Then the answer, the knowing, seemed to fill my mind. It was as if a switch had been thrown and the information had appeared for me to digest.

We are not *only* human or what we call human, we are something else. Sometimes humans exist without one of us inside their bodies. This is because we are a race of beings that on Earth we call 'spirit' and we spirits live inside this host body that would be, without us, essentially an animal. We call the combination 'human'. We are the product of two awareness's living inside one body. The body is just a shell.

This is why we sometimes struggle with ourselves, and why some of us have sought to annihilate great swathes of humanity. Being spirit does not mean that you are fully developed. Being human means you are developing. The very young souls need a place to go, to grow and to learn.

Welcome to kindergarten.

You are usually here on Earth so that you will learn to develop into something more. Becoming human is a fast way to increase your development as a spirit, but that also means that Earth and the other planets we go to, are often full of souls who have not lived many lives, so they are young souls. We have many souls on Earth who are working through issues of anger or discomfort with other emotions. In other words, there are many young souls on Earth and the young are often reckless or foolish. If you are an old or wise soul, your task is to steer the young ones away from their natural fecklessness.

Being given a body to live in also gives you different insights that as a spirit we do not have. You learn different lessons on Earth, lessons about the value of a physical body and respect for other people's needs and wants, because here, everything is limited. In the body we are like Robinson Crusoe. In spirit, there is no limit to space, abundance or time.

One other really valuable lesson from having a body is that we die, so every moment matters, as each moment could be your last one on Earth. I know that I want to make my mark, I want to be remembered for being a good soul, for helping, for loving, for being a friend, to my family, my peers and to the earth.

These thoughts, these knowings settled into my brain and I resumed observing my spiritual body. I was still aware of my physical body being attended to, but in an absent way. I had no idea how long I had been dead for now and I was disorientated and unsure of what I was supposed to do in Heaven. Should I be walking, looking for someone to help me, or wait where I was until someone came to collect me?

Feeling uncertain, I decided to wait where I was a little while longer. I finally got around to noticing that I was dressed; I was wearing striped cotton like pants. They were comfortable, loose and beautifully coloured. They looked as if they were made out of all the colours of the auric field, luminescent in their colour and arrangement. My top was purple.

A crowd of people stood near me, but I had yet not been noticed by them until now.

I felt quite comfortable standing there, observing this crowd. I did not feel the need to join them, nor did I feel left out by them. But as I kept thinking about where I was and what I should do, the knowledge that no-one was going to come and collect me, or help me sort things out came to me very clearly. Obviously, I was on my own. I was in Heaven, I was part of the community and I was essentially expected to cope. If I had listed my expectations of what heaven would be like and what I would experience when I arrived, being left to my own devices, to work things out and cope, was not one of those expectations. This knowledge was neither good nor bad. I did not feel hard done by, or excluded. It is a different feeling to anything you may feel on earth, but it was also not the embracing, warm, accepting feeling of love that I had assumed that I would experience.

As I played with my thoughts, and thought about a few things, I was shown that everything that was happening to me seemed to be directed by my thoughts: everything that happened to me depended on where I placed my attention. If I needed time to be calm and to think, I had that time. Thoughts were indeed things, and I could move and travel through this new location, just by thinking. But I could also feel that my thoughts were private: I shared what I wanted to share.

Right now I just needed time to adjust to where I was. Observe the stars, feel my body, look around.

But if I had been panicking or desperate, people would no doubt have come to collect me and help me.

So I stood still for a while. I did not feel the pressure to be anywhere, nor did I feel out of place, or uncomfortable. I was just content to be.

I focused on my locale trying to see if there was an obvious place to go to; something with a big sign with 'God this way' written on it, or something like that, but where I was just seemed to be a pleasant oasis with trees and plants around the place. I could see a mountain off in the distance, to the left of me and more trees in front of me. It felt like the space behind me was a drop of some sort, a cliff, or something like that. There was nothing outstanding here, it was just pleasant place. I saw no buildings, or crystal palaces, nothing that was outstanding.

It felt like this place that I was standing in, was a 'platform' of infinite size. This 'platform' seemed vast and was also 'floating', as if it was unattached to anything. It didn't seem to have any particular attachment to any location. Although I wondered if my thoughts were creating this location, it was as real to me as any Earth location, so even if this place was all some kind of fiction, it was pretty fine fiction.

What this place most seemed like to me was a meeting place where everybody could meet without necessarily staying here. People, beings, were walking around, moving, or even just resting. These beings were all clearly humanoid, but not all were 'human'. There were also animals but not as many animals as there were humanoids. Some of these beings were clustered together, talking. Others were sitting alone, waiting I suppose, for something. There did not seem to be any sort of fashion that I could identify. No one was in clothing that resembled clothes from the 50's or 60's, or the medieval times. No one was dressed like a hippy, or an Indian or a Japanese person. Everybody just seemed to be in comfortable, nondescript clothes that seemed to reflect different colours, constantly.

All of this assessing and summing up of where I was, and my situation, happened very quickly. What takes some time for me to write, and for you to read, was, in Heaven's reality, very quick.

Then I decided that I was ready to meet other beings.

I suddenly became very worried about my body, hoping and trusting that it was being looked after by Bernie. And just as suddenly I was back in my bedroom.

...Stepping through...

My room was even fuller than before, with many people in there. I noticed that my body was now on the floor and that there were three firemen in the room as well as Bernie. One of the firemen, was kneeling behind my head and two of them were kneeling beside me. Bernie was still on the bed and it was to him that I looked. Interestingly, he looked right at the place where I was, then he looked away again, as if his vision had slipped off me, as if he had 'seen' me, but been unable to believe it. Bernie looked down at my body and I could see the concern in his face and *feel* the concern in his heart. His heart felt like cold, grey concrete.

I realized that the firemen were about to shock my body and I did not want to watch that, not because it would have hurt me, but because it would be unnecessary for me to see. I had other things I wanted to do whilst they were working on me. I turned my mind away and I was back in Heaven.

Immediately it felt like the ground rolled beneath me. I reached out to grasp anything that I could that would help me steady myself, but before I found purchase, I was fine again. I realized that it was the shock passing through me that I had felt. Each further time that they shocked me I felt a similar feeling go through my spiritual body. The connection to my physical body, although it was decreasing, would cause an imbalance in my spiritual body each time they pumped a strong electric shock through it.

By now I was aware that even if I made it back alive, my brain would most likely be damaged. It was a constant stream of concern that was underlying everything else. I wanted to relax and be fully present in this place where I was, but I knew that if I did that, I *would* be dead. Unable to do anything immediately about my circumstances, I started walking and looking around me, trying to remember what details I could.

Heaven felt vast, but also felt contained. It could stretch out to be as big as necessary, but it could also be as small as needed. The size seemed to change in my perception, sometimes for no reason that I could ascertain. I also knew that there were other places that I had not yet seen; that this Heaven suited me and what I needed, right now. Because it was an energetic place, not physical as we are, it could move and alter to suit my perceptions. I also knew that it *was* a physical place in that it was constructed of electromagnetic energy and that natural laws would apply to it. It was just that we did not know what the natural laws were, necessarily. For instance, if I wanted to go into another time in our Earth reality, I would have to do so as a spirit, a ghost, or a body. As a ghost, I would have limited contact with humans and very little of that contact is a healthy contact – people would more be afraid of me. As a spiritual guide I could have greater contact in terms of helpfulness, but I would never truly be visible. It would take me longer to reach that level of a guide.

But as a being with a physical body, I would have opportunity to have the greatest impact, but that impact would require limiting me, defining myself with a physical body, making myself vulnerable to emotional pain and loss and relinquishing my mental capacity. I would not be as smart, or as wise.

The knowledge that I now had in Heaven and was able to use, in both Heaven and on Earth, I had gained through great personal expense by being corporeal. The pain of being human gained me wisdom as a spirit.

I had thought that when I died, all the knowledge I needed would be given back to me, that I would remember all my past lives, my purpose from this life, that I would have an ease inside of me once more. I wasn't disappointed to realize that this was not the case, but I was a little surprised. It seemed that if Heaven was created by what I expected, then I knew very little about what I expected. Heaven was very different to anything I had imagined and I certainly felt completely differently to anything I had expected to feel.

I had assumed that in Heaven all my problems would be gone. That I would be happy and at peace and that all my 'silly' feelings would be gone. I was wrong. I could see everything from a different perspective, but I still felt the same feelings. I was like a cartographer, charting the whole region rather than being the traveller making the journey. I knew that I still had to come to a peaceful place with my feelings, whether in Heaven or on Earth.

The place in Heaven where I currently was - was where you go when you are refreshing and renewing from a physical life. This is where choices were made by you and for you. It was only when this choice was final that you would be able to connect with beings like your guides.

I came to understand that many beings find life on the planets difficult and so they needed to time to recover. It seemed like 'living' a corporeal existence was a bit like being in a boxing match. Hard work and often painful, but the rewards outweighed the pain.

I also came to understand that because Heaven was literally everywhere, even though it was in a different dimension, that time travel and space travel was very possible, just by being in heaven. To go to another planet, you step *through* Heaven and onto that planet, same with time travel, so you may have lived in this age, being born in 1959, for instance, but next time you live you may be in 1781, or 2398. It made no difference to Heaven. It was all there already and just waiting for the players to put on the masks. Time is not fixed. You can move to anywhere and to anytime that suits you. If you connect with someone, it is absolutely brilliant that you found each other. Of all the places, times and planets that you could be, you are both right here, right now.

We, humankind, seek travel amongst the stars because that is our 'soul right' and even though, now we are in physical, and we have forgotten that we were once spirit, when we are in spirit again, we will remember. In spirit our brains are limitless, but they have real restrictions in human form. We have to sacrifice memory for the ability to learn and have fun in the flesh. We come to Earth and the other planets that we occupy, to experience food, sex and roller coaster rides. It is the fast track, but it is not without cost.

And part of the cost is our intellect. Because we have a limited brain space, we need to relinquish the memories of past lives and of Heaven to live as a human. And after all, we are here to learn to be human, as we are already a fully developed spirit.

But going outwards is often easier than going inward. For instance, we can stretch out to the stars more easily than going to the depths of the ocean, which is a much harder place to traverse. Likewise, it is usually easier to see someone else's problem, than it is to see your own.

With all these thoughts in my mind, I knew that I needed to move on further. I had decided that I wanted to find God so that I could plead my case. I was also starting to feel concern at how long I had seemed to be gone. The sky around me was still dark though, and I took that as a good sign.

In the far distance, I could see the mountain that I had spotted earlier, and now I realized that there was also a light crowning the mountain; I 'knew' that this light was God: the being that I *called* God. This vast energy, which is beyond human, is as bright as the sun, but was gentler on the eyes than the sun is. The sun hurts to look at, whereas this energy source was bright, but calming. As with the sun though, we can't get too close to it, without being destroyed, yet we can look at this light without hurting our eyes.

Information about God/Source flooded into me as my memories were restored. God is not male, nor female. It is not patriarchal, nor the Goddess, nor the horned devil or any of these concepts, nor is it none of these concepts. God would not demand celibacy or female circumcision or the decision to not eat meat, ride bicycles, or that we 'worship' anything. God does not require blood sacrifice to survive. God does not have just one world or only white males in service to the Source.

God/Source is everything, everybody, everywhere. It is every thought, every belief, and every notion no matter how crazy because we, us, all of us, create God/Source. Some people or cultures choose to worship a part of it, which would be like worshipping the arms of the human body, or the stomach.

In the end we are sent out as explorers, sending telegrams home for the delight of God and all to enjoy. Our experience is the experience of all.

That which is God is energy Source; vast, information hungry, peaceful and curious energy source made up of thousands, millions, billions of spirits from this planet and other planets. God does not have a grand scheme for you or me, but God has knowledge and compassion and interest. God is a benign parent who wants you to have fun and to enjoy yourself. You only live *this* life once. Fortunately, you will have thousands of one life's.

My quest, my need to find God continued to grow in me. I was aware that my body back in my bedroom was physical and did have a finite time frame, so I continued on towards the mountain, determined to find someone who could give me answers.

As I walked on towards the mountain, I could also see beings around me who felt quite different to 'human' souls, even alien human souls. As I was pondering over them I realized that they were angels. Looking at them I 'knew' that angels act as transformers: they pass the God energy through them so that we can communicate with that energy. This is why angels are here, different to us yet helping us. When you are speaking to angels you *are* speaking to God, as much as you are able to.

If you spoke to God with nothing in between you and God, you would rejoin to God and no longer be separate. We are all a part of God. It would not destroy you, but 'you' would be lost.

Quickly I moved closer to the angels and towards the mountain, reasoning that where they were, God was more likely to be. I hoped.

I stopped and I smiled, feeling relief, when I recognized a tall man heading towards me. This man looked like a desert dweller. I had previously met this man during my near death experience when I was four years old and I know that it was Jesus. He stopped as I continued to walk but he was clearly waiting for me, standing patiently with a few other beings standing behind him and around him. I almost started to sing with joy when I realized that the beings standing behind Jesus were my guides, but my focus was entirely on Jesus.

"Hello Carmel," Jesus smiled, as he walked toward me. "Welcome home," he smiled again, welcoming me to him, his arms held open.

Jesus and the things you talk about

Jesus appeared to me as a well built and capable man. He was slender – not heavy set – much as you would expect someone who walked many miles a day to look. He seemed in appearance to be about 35-years-old. He was a man in his prime. He had mid brown, wavy hair and dark blue eyes, with a beard and moustache. He was wearing a simple, homespun robe and his arms had the sinewy look about them of a person who was well used to hard manual labour. He looked and he exuded both capability and confidence. I stepped forward and into his arms. I could feel him enfolding me, and then my Guides were also there.

I remember feeling intense joy as my guides, Peter, Hiram, Rondor and Alexander clustered around me. We mingled and hugged, with me laughing and crying at the same time. I did not know if I was joyous at being in Heaven, sad at the life I had left behind, scared at what I was seeing in heaven; angry at the trials I had been through on earth. There was no peace inside me and that was the strongest feeling – a deep sense of a lack of peace and what I needed, what I craved, was peace.

"You have done very well; you achieved what we wanted you to do with your life," Jesus spoke; I looked at him quizzically "You successfully brought Metatron's energy into the world. Now it's time for you to be with us again." Jesus smiled once more, indicating the space around him. It was obvious that this was my home and I was welcome here.

I had felt overwhelmed with emotion as soon as Jesus began to speak. I really did not know what I wanted to do. I hopped from foot to foot and felt about 12-years-old and probably also felt pretty stupid. I wanted to yell at him and hug him and just cry and cry. I wanted to return to Earth and keep on with my work and I also just wanted to be told that there was nothing else for me to do in that regard. Jesus smiled at me and I stepped forward into his arms. I was home. All the years of pain that I had felt, all the disappointments, all the hurts, all the angst, seemed to disappear in that moment. Every moment of hurt and pain and loneliness melted as I cried and cried whilst Jesus held me.

After a while I felt calm again and Jesus let me go. Then Jesus and I sat together quietly, on the grass, at the base of a palm tree. Peter, Hiram, Rondor and Alexander also sat with us.

At first I had nothing to say, I just wanted to feel what I was feeling. But I knew I had many questions and I started to ask them, without hesitation. I asked questions like, 'Why am I here? Why does it hurt so much? Why are people unkind? Is money wrong? Is suicide wrong? Sleeping with lots of people wrong? I would like to think that everything I asked was deep and meaningful questions, but the truth is, I asked what weighed on my mind. I asked what weighs on the mind of everybody who is living. Perhaps you would like to think that I had not left behind the being that was Carmel and perhaps I should have asked deep questions like 'How do we fix world poverty?' but I didn't ask that. I know the answer to that already. We can't. Life is not fair, which is how we learn. We are *here* to experience unfairness, rage, love, kindness, hurt, betrayal and other emotions. How can Heaven rob us of all that we asked to feel?

I asked questions that Carmel would have asked, because that is who I was. Whether it was under this name or another name, the soul was the same soul.

This is my conversation with Jesus, as best as I can remember it.

We, Jesus and I, sat together at the base of a palm tree, on grass. We were facing each other and Jesus had his legs crossed. My guides stayed with us. I could feel them and their protectiveness of me. I could feel that they wanted to speak to me and in the back of my mind I wondered why they did not. I could also feel that there were Angels close by.

"Are you the son of God, really?"

"I am." Jesus said simply. "I am the 'child' of That Which Is. I am part of That Which Is."

"Am I?"

"You are also a part of That Which Is." I looked at Jesus quietly, waiting for more.

"That Which Is," he continued "Is billions of souls, all together. That Which Is *cannot* be one Being, one man, one woman, one child. That Which Is cannot be one. It is many. You are part of that many that has chosen to be separate from One. You also are not a man, nor a woman, but are both and neither. You are human and not human. Spirit and not spirit. You are part of that many that has chosen to be separate."

"Does my being separate upset That Which Is?"

"No. It does not. You have not left. You are not gone. You have separated just as a child separates from you. You are living your soul's desire and that makes That Which Is content. In fact," Jesus continued his explanation, "You being separate helps That Which Is understand this Universe." Jesus indicated the space all around us.

I shook my head, puzzled. "Is there is only one Universe?"

Jesus laughed. "There are many Universes."

"That Which Is knows everything already?"

Jesus shook his head "That Which Is knows everything, but which part of that Everything are you? Which will you be in this lifetime? What happiness will you earn, what love will you give? What choices will you make? The choices you make are what create the Energy that runs the Universe. You are an energy being. Everything is connected and every moment matters. No moment is more or less than any other. I see one day you will write these words. One day another soul will read these words and they will see in them much more than you realized you were placing there. That Which Is would like to know which ripple you have created. What will come from these words we have spoken and where will they go? You have created far more than you realize."

I was fascinated by his words. So many images accompanied them that I was amazed. I was shown a constant diorama of people reading these explanations by Jesus and some of these people being given hope, others deciding to create something from the feelings this inspired and yet others just walking away, battling the urge to do something with how they felt. We all respond differently.

My questions continued...

"So what I do matters to That Which Is?"

"Yes, it matters very much that you breathe and create. You are creating this Universe and That Which Is is the centre of this Universe."

"Why was I there, on earth?"

"We asked you to be there. Sometimes That Which Is wants more known than is already known. So many souls had asked for Energy to complete them, to make their journey more fulfilled that we asked you to carry it for us," In my mind I could see an image like an Olympic torch being passed from soul to soul over the centuries. A long time is a quick time in spirit. This had been a plan, and I, my body, had been centuries in the making, growing and breeding into a being that could pass on Metatronic Energy to other people. I was the end product of a long line of energy transmitters.

In one part of me I felt happy to have been able to help. It is not that my role was anymore, or any less important than anyone else's role. It was just a path that I and That Which Is had agreed to.

But there was another part of me that called out 'What about my life? What about what I wanted!' I had always known that I was driven. Now I could see the fullness of why I was driven. It was part of the reason for the despair that I had felt before I died.

Having been to Heaven and now come back, I believe that That Which Is called me home so that I could come back and live as a human, choosing consciously to pass this energy and this message on, rather than doing this work because I felt called to it. Although it may sound terrible to have died, it gave me an opportunity to decide that I wanted to live, and *how* I wanted to live, consciously and as a human, with a clear memory of that decision.

"So every thought that I have, every rotten idea, angry retort, unfulfilled plan...?"

"All matter to That Which Is. All is heard. Every request is answered. Every moment is noticed, Carmel, but no judgement is given to any moment. It is your life and you are free to live it as you could have walked away from our request to you for help."

I realized then that although I had been driven to be a Medical Intuitive, it had also made it my passion. I was happy when I was doing it and not happy when I was not.

"It has been a long journey," I sighed.

"Very long. You have been many lifetimes in the making."

I could feel myself starting to cry again, overwhelmed with the feelings that I was experiencing but I knew that I had limited time. Sorrow was for when I had the luxury of time.

I put my feelings aside and continued my questions. "Why does it hurt so much for me to be human?"

"You were 'made' to feel people's emotions and to recognize what they are feeling. That is part of your gift." I put that aside for now.

"Why are people unkind?"

"People are unkind because other people or events make them feel unbalanced or curious. When people are off balance, they often strike out at what they believe they are afraid of. Remember that many souls on the Earth are very young. On each planet there is a mixture of young souls and old souls so that the young souls will have someone there to help them to learn. Young souls are also very full of joy, but often quick to react to circumstances that make them uncomfortable. How kind were you when you were young in spirit?"

I remembered scenes from other lives. Often I was not very kind.

"Is money wrong?"

"No, money is not wrong. It is an energy source and how you use it may be wrong. But having money is not wrong. However, you may have chosen a lifetime with no money because you wish to be reminded of what it is like to struggle to find that energy. When people suffer a lack, they seek to fill it and often they hurt themselves very much by seeking that energy."

"Is sex with a lot of people wrong? I mean, are we meant to marry one person and only have sex with them?"

"Sex is not wrong. Letting the wrong energy into your being is unkindness to you. The wounds to the body will heal quickly, but the wounds to your soul take longer to repair. Any action that harms your body is against yourself. It is against the agreement you made with that body. You are the judge of that action."

I was concerned that I would regret asking all these 'stupid' questions. I remember thinking to myself 'I bet I am the only person who has asked such dumb, unspiritual questions.' But you know what? I doubt it. I think that when we all get to Heaven, we are all of us more concerned with the life just gone than in any higher purpose, which is why we are not quickly reborn.

As Oscar Wilde said "We are all of us in the gutter, but some of us are looking at the stars."

On Earth, when you are in your physical body you can ask just one question at a time, but when you're in spirit, you can ask many questions and have them answered simultaneously. It's as if you're uploading the questions and downloading the answers, right into your spiritual brain, just as if you were interacting with a powerful computer. Because your mentality does not have the limiting case of a brain, you are intellectually unlimited. Later, I came to understand that although I had all this information, whether I chose to use it or not, or even to remember it, depended on me and my own intention.

While I was speaking with Jesus, he and I also discussed my life just passed, and my work as a Medical Intuitive, using Metatronic Energy.

It dawned on me that Jesus was telling me that the Carmel Bell life was finished – I would now go on, in spirit, to a new life. This was my 'life review', such as it was. I felt shocked. My life seemed so small. It had seemed so lonely and unhappy, with too many challenges. I have faced cancer, a brain tumour, rape, rejection, and more. It had often felt like too many tragedies but as a Medical Intuitive I had learned that each crisis was of my own making and was my own responsibility. This realisation did not excuse anyone else of their bad behaviour or let them off the hook, but learning this truth had, in my life as 'Carmel Bell', allowed me to forgive them and to forgive me for doing this to myself and my life. This truth had given me back my responsibility and my power. After all, each hurt that you cause to someone else you also do to yourself. There was no need for me to be angry anymore, or bitter.

But I wanted to have a chance to be back on Earth, being happy and having fun before I died. And to do that, I needed to convince Jesus.

In Heaven, as I underwent my life review I was pleased to learn that what I had thought I was doing, I really had been doing. I had spent my life helping other people, being as kind as I could be, in the way that I wanted to be. Not following anyone else's path, not doing as I was told, not being afraid to stand by my beliefs, but being kind to others, treating them well, whilst I tried to treat me well, also. The hardest person to be kind to is often you. The secret really is that you are here to live your life, no-one else's. If it makes you *un*happy, don't do it. If you are unsure or if everything makes you unhappy, work it through until you are happy. The source of my unhappiness has often been other people's attitudes towards me when I did not fulfil their expectations. Sometimes it was their fear of me because I was different or they were afraid I would see things that they did not want me to see.

A lot of people who were regarded as 'normal' had an uncomfortable feeling when they were around me. They thought that I would 'read' them, or preach to them, or suddenly grow a second head. But I think that I often attracted these people because I needed to be challenged on my belief that what I was doing with Medical Intuition was odd. This secret fear/belief made me unhappy with me. These people were just signposting that to me.

It is like when you see an unguarded photo of yourself and you say to yourself 'Do I really look like that?' Kind of amazed, kind of proud, sometimes pleased, but more often than not, dismayed that someone caught a picture of you that did not fit in with your idea of you. Your 'bad side' as it were. I felt like a lot of my bad side had been put on display. Because my life was probably destined to be more public than usual, all my points, both good and bad, were there for all to see. It felt like I was living in a fish bowl, never free and I was uncomfortable.

But often years later, you will see that photo again and you will realize that it was not such a bad picture after all. That it really did look like you. I felt like that now. Caught out, but not ashamed of it.

"So what is the meaning of life? To be rich, famous, or sacrificial?"

Jesus laughed quite loudly. "It is to learn how to treat other souls. You are on Earth to interact closely with other souls."

I admit I felt a little dismayed by this answer. Dismay was my most immediate response. I wanted to be given the deepest secret of the Universe, something like 'The meaning of life, the reason you are all on Earth doing this, is to learn to transform your energy system into pure energy, overcome the need to eat, sleep, laugh. Put aside all urges that are considered base, and be able to fly, flapping your arms only, from here to Moscow, without needing refuelling once!'

I wanted to *understand* what it was all really about. Something, anything, that could give me a heads up, instead of being told that what I was already doing was what I should be doing.

I was kind to people not because I had to be, or because I was afraid to not be, but because that was how I wanted to be. I had learned how to treat other people properly throughout my life. That did not mean that I never felt hurt, jealous, angry or sad. I was human, after all, but it did mean that I had learned to not act on those feelings; to consider others before I rushed off and did something foolish.

"Have I ever been free?"

"Yes. You were asked if you would do this for us all and you agreed. The choice was yours,"

"But every day since then has been me doing this task for Heaven?

"That's right, but you were still free."

"You let Bernie come to be with me, help me?" Jesus nodded again, "Then let me go back to be with him!" I was distressed at realising that I was expected to stay here. I wasn't ready to let go of me or my life with Bernie.

I knew the pain that Bernie would suffer if I died. He had many years to live and he would live those years totally alone. As we had talked I had been seeing a vision of the future and Jesus had shown me some of the future for Bernie. "I want to go back!" I insisted. "Please!"

"Your task is completed." Jesus told me quietly. I had been aware that there was another being there with us whilst Jesus and I talked, but I had been focussed solely on Jesus and my desire to return to Earth.

"I was too human!" I complained 'It hurt too much."

Jesus laughed softly. "You were there *to be* human. You are *already* a spirit. As a human you need to eat, drink, love, play, have sex, *join* with people. As a spirit you, we, are often more solitary."

I thought of all the times that I had carelessly done things, said things, or been angry. I knew that I had never hurt or maimed anything or anyone deliberately, but I was curious, puzzled and a little prepared to be upset. Everyone had always told me that I was on Earth to be as spiritual as possible and this had never made sense to me. Here I was in Heaven, being told that what I had thought was correct, that we are here on Earth to be *human* and I was *feeling upset* about that!

"You must not try to be spirit when you are in human form. You must be the best human you can be. Laugh, cry, love, be kind, because it is not easy to be those things. It is a choice and making the right choice can be hard. For a person who has never felt temptation, the thought of being tempted is nothing. This is the reason why you go to each life without memory of your past lives, without certain knowledge of another place. So that you *are* free to be human. You can only base your choice on the time you are in and the place you are dwelling." Jesus looked at me. "There is no second chance in your life as a human. You are only the choices you make."

This made sense to me. I thought of all the people who tried to ignore their own lives, their own families in the interest of being as 'spiritual' as possible. If they were here on Earth to be a spirit, they would not have taken a body. "Does that mean that it truly does not matter what I do? What anybody does?"

"It matters very much. Every moment matters. Your choices are you, and you are defined by your choices. Where you go from here will be decided by the choices you made on Earth."

"So is murder wrong?"

"Of course. Murder is wrong. It pains your heart and stops you from being the person you were meant to be, as well as taking from the victim their right to choose." Jesus looked at me. 'You live in your heart, Carmel. Follow it, as it holds a map to what you want to do and who you want to be. Your heart cannot lie."

"Mine stopped!"

"Yours was broken. We brought you home to mend you."

"But why?" I cried softly. I felt like a pendulum, swinging between one emotion to the next. Fear, happiness, frustration, I was confused.

"Always when you feel different from those around you, your heart will suffer. Your heart bears the pain."

"I thought we were all the same." I cried

"We are not all the same. We are all growing at different rates and there must be those who lead and those who walk the path behind them. You had a task and it was hard. We asked you to do this for us, and you agreed. Do you remember?"

My mind flew back to the first time I had died, when I was four, "I think so, but I didn't know it would be so hard and then give me back so little!" I was being honest. I had hoped for more from the life that I had led. More happiness, more peace, more contentment and yet, "I want to go back!" I said again. I was so scared of returning and yet I could not stay.

"Your task is completed and you are here now. There are others who can continue for you."

"I don't want to be here!" I insisted, "Not yet, not now. Bernie needs me."

Jesus remained calm and I felt like I was becoming more and more distressed. I did not know how to convince him that I could do this. I could be happy; I could find peace in a human life. I wanted a chance to be back on Earth and having fun. I wanted a chance to learn to be comfortable enough with me that I did not feel judged. I knew that now was the time in my life when I did actually stand a chance of living a life for me.

I realized that this discussion with Jesus was my life review. I was pleased to realize that I had actually been doing on earth what I thought I had been doing. Whilst Jesus and I had been speaking I could also see a constant stream of memories, reviewing my life, from birth, to now. All the great things I had accomplished, all my successes, my kindnesses, the fun that I had experienced. Laughing, dancing, playing, loving. As well, all the negative things were shown to me. All the times that I had been unnecessarily cruel, or thoughtless, I was shown. Opportunities that I had walked by, to do the right thing, say the right thing. Even times when people had been kind to me and I had rejected their kindness because I was feeling hurt or for some other reason. All these moments had either hurt me, or helped me. No moment was unimportant and each one had been stored in my body, in the cells of my body and in my DNA and had also been passed on to my children.

Also, whilst I was speaking with Jesus, I occasionally switched my attention back to my body in my bedroom at home, checking on what was happening. I did this as easily as you'd change channels on a TV set, although I was aware of both places at the same time.

I was aware of the firemen and paramedics working on my body. The fireman who was holding the oxygen mask suddenly looked up at me, right where I was and caught my attention. I moved closer to him, placing my nose almost on his nose. "I will remember you," I whispered. Weeks later, when I went to meet the firemen who had helped to save me, I did remember him. I walked right up to this fireman and looked him in the face. "I remember you," I said.

While I felt relief to see that my body was still being worked on by the paramedics I also knew that it meant that I still had time to argue my case. I knew when they gave me a shock because I could feel the energy disruption to my being, but I also knew that it was becoming less likely that I would be revived because the effect was decreasing on me in Heaven. I turned my attention back to Heaven. I needed to convince Jesus to let me go back or I was dead.

"I want to speak to God!" I told Jesus. "That Which Is, let me speak to him please."

"You cannot," he shook his head as he insisted; 'It is not that I say you may not. I am saying that you cannot."

The other being, the angel, who was standing with Jesus and I moved forward then, into my 'attention' space. I could tell that this being was an angel, not because 'he' had wings, because 'he' did not, but because the energy around him was so strong and so bright compared to mine and to Jesus' energy. I was fascinated. It was very different to ours. It was more luminescent in tone and if it had been a music note, it probably would have sounded sweet and resonant.

"You asked to come home," this being explained to me.

"Who are you?"

The angel spoke. "I am Metatron,"

"Noah was a drunk. Look what he accomplished." Metatron in Dogma

"I remember you!" I jumped to my feet and walked forward towards Metatron. I looked at Metatron in amazement as memories of my previous NDE came flooding clearly back to me. I remembered being four years old and dying briefly from shock after I had been burnt when my nightgown had caught on fire.

I also remembered all the other times that Metatron had had a hand in my life. There were so many ways that he had touched my world.

Now I'm standing in Heaven again but this time I am in Heaven 'proper' and not the waiting room. I know that I am in a precarious situation. I am aware that time is running out for me. Even though I was out of my body, I could still only describe it as being aware of my body. I knew that it was in trouble. I could feel all the emotions from my first NDE still hitting me and I knew the full impact that that experience had had on me.

Suddenly, standing in Heaven, all the hurts of the past years came barrelling down on me. I could have drowned in the weight of all the grief and the disappointment I have felt. I could hardly breathe and a small part of my brain noticed how ironic that this was – that even though I was not breathing and I had no heart to beat, I could still feel breathless, I could still feel my heart breaking in my chest. All the moments that I was hurt, or hurt, felt ashamed, missed the point, did not see or chose not to see. I felt at a loss, crushed, a failure.

Stunned, overwhelmed, I retreated. In Heaven I fell to my knees, tears streaking down my face, but another part of me stepped through the dimensions back to my body. Back on Earth I was aware of a shock jolting my body. I watched my body arch, I could see the electricity arcing through me and I knew that it would not work. My heart was broken.

I could feel Bernie's emotions; hope and then despair. I could feel his heart growing 'denser' with each passing minute. I knew that this was a pain he would not recover from in this lifetime. Bernie has resilience greater than almost anyone I know, but losing me would have been too much. This was no better than what I had just fled. I turned around, and feeling quite odd, I stepped back through.

And back into my body on the ground in heaven, where no-one but me had placed me. Holding onto the grief of this life and countless other lives had brought me to my knees. I struggled to my feet again. "I want to speak to God." I looked at Metatron. I walked past Jesus and right up to Metatron. "I want to speak to God!" I repeated. I felt angry, but almost as soon as I had spoken the words, the anger bled away. I realized that anger was just a protection from emotions that were too strong for us to cope with.

"You cannot," he shook his head. The compassion, the love that I could feel flow from Metatron almost crushed me. I wanted no softness. I wanted God. I wanted to find out why I was angry and hurt. Angels are taller and larger than we are and I had to look up at Metatron. I could tell you also that he had hair and shoulders and arms and legs. He wore similar robes to what I could see on Jesus. But I cannot remember precise details of hair colour or skin colour or nose shape. It feels that each time I looked at him he would appear in the most pleasing of forms for me, or the form which I could most accept. I can remember that staring into his eyes was like drowning in pools of endless emotions. Staring into his face was like looking into something that was me, and so much more than me, staring into the mirror and seeing your own eyes and being startled at the compassion for yourself that you see staring back at you.

Metatron carried in him every emotion that I had ever felt, every grief, every joy, every moment and he did something with them, these emotions. I think he gave them to what we call God. No emotion, no love, no pain is ever forgotten. It is carried and stored in heaven.

I pulled myself out of his space and asked "Why not?"

I was thinking to myself, *'Why can't I speak to God? What's wrong with me?'* Yet another hurt, yet another judgment. When would I be good enough?

Metatron shook his head, "That Which Is" he explained "loves you and because That Which Is loves you, you cannot speak to That Which Is yet." I knew again, with absolute certainty, that we were all speaking in another language, one that I had never heard on Earth before, but one that we were all speaking, even the animals. This language was passed telepathically and with it came the emotions and the intent that you felt with it. I knew, I recognized, that this is a skill that I also have on Earth, which is why I am so good at telling what people actually meant and also who was telling me the truth, or lying to me.

With the skill of telepathy also came implicit understanding and I knew that the word that I used for God translated into "That Which Is" or 'Everything and Everybody'. With it came an image into my mind of billions of intertwined souls, wrapped together, moving together, growing together out of the actions of all of us on Earth and other planets.

In Heaven there is only one language and we all speak it/hear it. Even the animals speak this language.

There is also only one faith/belief/knowledge and all religions are part of that one faith/belief/knowledge, but only one part, not the complete whole. Whether you were Jewish, or Muslim or Christian, you were neither right, nor wrong. We are all one. This is knowledge that you just 'have', you do not need to ask it, once your

Spirit is back again with all that is there. Each of us brings with us to Earth a small part of what we know from Heaven, but usually not enough of the knowledge, or with enough clarity for it to be thought of as the complete truth.

Even me, writing this, there are parts that I have forgotten, and other parts that belong only to me and there were often three or four different conversations happening at once. On Earth, we will never know Heaven.

Metatron continued speaking. "If you come too close to That Which Is, in this form, you would cease to exist as you. You would rejoin with That Which Is. To remain separate it is through me that you must speak." I was silent for a few moments after he finished speaking. I wanted time to digest his words and the feelings that he had conveyed with them. On Earth a word is a word. In Heaven a word is a feeling and a word. Communication is both faster and more meaningful in Heaven because you feel the weight of the words and all the meanings of them. As spirit, there is no barrier between us and the meaning that we intend. As I look back over what I spoke about, I sometimes struggle with how moralistic it sounds, but if heard with the feeling, the intent, behind it, you soon realize that so much comes with the words that it all makes sense.

These beings are not judging us. God – That Which Is – is not judging us. They feel our humanity and relish it. They feel compassion for the struggle that we go through so that we can send knowledge from Earth to Heaven. This life is not an easy journey. It is quite hard to be human.

Metatron, Jesus and I sat down together and began to 'feel' each other as we spoke. I knew what we were doing. We were exchanging energy. We do this on Earth as well, but we do not recognize it for what it is, but it is this energy exchange that allows healings from energy be performed. The single biggest blocker of this kind of energy work is fear – any kind of fear. Fear of the illness; fear of the future, past – anything. This is why anxiety panic disorder is one of the most destructive illnesses to the human body. It creates huge stores of fear in the energy system.

I remembered the stories that had been taught to me from the Christian Bible, of how Metatron was the 'Voice of God' and how he spoke for God. I remembered that Metatron had been human once and had been taken to Heaven and made into an angel so that we humans could speak to God safely.

Metatron was as close to God as we could traverse, without being reabsorbed into source. We would each of us reunite with God, when we had finished our growth journey. We are a flame that has broken away from the bright burning light of That Which Is.

Metatron, Jesus and I sat together, on the ground of Heaven, a tree at our back - the same tree that had been with us when I died when I was four. It was a palm tree. I don't know why it was a palm tree but I do know that whenever I see a palm tree I feel a world of infinite possibilities.

I was silent for a few moments, thinking to myself 'This is the last chance I might get. Be smart, Carmel, be smart.' There were so many questions that I wanted to ask.

I asked Metatron if I was teaching his energy as he wanted it taught. I asked him if it was even okay for me to be teaching it. I asked why I felt lonely and he told me because I was aware that I was disconnected from heaven. He explained that I was highly energy sensitive I was aware of my absence from Heaven.

I spoke to him about my work on Earth, using the energy that he channeled to me and he told me that he had been happy with what I had done. He affirmed for me that they had asked me to do this for them, so although it had been my choice to say 'yes' or 'no', I had felt driven to complete my task once I had become human.

I had been reluctant to come back to Earth this last lifetime, and I had known the task would be an almost impossible mission, yet it was asked of me. And yet I said yes. Now I was in Heaven, feeling like a failure.

"They weren't ready yet!" I complained to Metatron. "I couldn't reach enough people! I couldn't get them to understand."

"They will be. You did not fail." Metatron assured me. "They had to first be ready to use this 'frequency'," He explained. "It is a higher vibration to those energies that have been used widely on Earth before,"

Into my mind flowed the concept of time, frequencies and an 'energy ladder'. What I, and others have been doing, as we introduced these different frequencies to the world was preparing the world to be able to absorb and utilize the higher frequencies. There are others like me out there; there are others like me in Australia.

We are infants still in energy use. Each step up the frequency ladder required time for a 'body adjustment' to be able to take place, but a body adjustment of the whole planet.

We, humans, are souls of an advanced species, residing in the bodies of a race of beings native to our Earth. We are inhabitants in a host body, and this is why we *are* able to go on and live other lives – many, many lives. As Nanci Danison put it in her book '*Backwards*', we are 'Light Being Souls inhabiting Human host animal bodies.'

The bodies that we now possess are as advanced as they are, over other animal's bodies, because of our presence in them. It could easily have been aardvarks that we chose to inhabit, or even slugs, but we chose apes. I would suspect because of the thumbs.

But when our body dies, we leave the body and we enter into Heaven where we rest, rejuvenate and get ready to come back for another round and a new body. We have been preparing these bodies as a species to accept higher frequencies. I will be intrigued to see what energy comes after this and what it can do.

Sometimes we come back very quickly and at other times we can take a long time to be ready. I was shown that the average length of time is a lifetime, so that you are not likely to meet your children, or your mother, for instance, from this lifetime.

Whilst I was still absorbing this new knowledge, Jesus spoke: "It's time," He said. All three of us stood up. I knew that he meant that it was time for me to go back to my body.

Jesus took my hands and looked into my eyes. Jesus and Metatron had agreed to let me return to Earth because of my not so subtle insistence. "Are you sure you want to return?" Jesus asked, somewhat compassionately. "It will be much harder than you realize. You will be hurt in ways you have never felt before. You will feel betrayal as well as many other disappointments. "

If I wanted to return, this was it. I could feel myself hesitate, just for a moment. If Jesus says it will be hard, I guess it will be and I was scared. They could feel my hesitation.

"If you don't go back now, the damage will be too great for you to repair," Jesus said.

I looked into the eyes of Jesus. There was no doubt left in my mind. Of course I would go back, but I could see the compassion in him, for me. We all make agreements before we're born, as to what we'll do with our time on earth. My initial contract for Carmel Bell had been fulfilled. I was now preparing to go back with no purpose, other than love.

Metatron stood at the shoulder of Jesus. I nodded to him.

"Can I do anything for you?" I asked them both.

"Yes, thank you, you can." Jesus smiled. "We will help you." And with that Jesus gave me a task that sounds simple but is feeling quite hard. "We want you to teach as many people as you can about Metatron's Energy." I nodded. Jesus continued "There is always a reason for what happens and a way out of the darkest of moments. You choose how you want to be. Remember that. It is your choice if you stay ill or heal." I could see a picture of me being brain damaged, still living, still helping Bernie to raise our children, but with no responsibilities, no college, no clinic. I knew that I could choose this if I wanted to. I did not.

With that message burning in my mind, I allowed all of me to step through the dimensions and to fully leave Heaven.

To leave Heaven was a matter of thinking about where I wanted to be and reaching for that place. It was not difficult to do. Just before I stepped through completely I turned and asked Jesus one last question.

"Star Trek," I asked Jesus, "Is it real? Does that happen?"

Jesus laughed. A great, loud laugh. "Yes, Carmel. It is real." My mind seemed to fill up with images, scenes, people and places from a future life – a life that I have already lived but have not yet reached. I saw myself seeing stars, reaching stars, moving into galaxies that I had never even heard of yet.

And I knew then that we succeed, against all odds, and against most expectations. Humanity will rise above the current state to grow beyond the narrowness of our own beliefs. We will not destroy this world; we will not make enemies amongst the stars. Mankind will prevail.

Chapter Eighteen:

Re-entry

I stepped through Heaven and back into my bedroom as simply as walking through my front door to return home. Then I quietly stood unseen in my room for a few moments, standing near my window and out of the way of all the other people in the room.

I looked around me. As I was standing over near my bedroom window I could not see my body immediately because it was on the floor, hidden by my bed and with quite a few people clustered around it.

I could see Bernie and three ambulance officers, as well as the three firemen who had been there from the start. The atmosphere in the room was grim and somber. I watched the scene for a few seconds, assessing the situation as the firemen around me started to slow down. The fireman at my head asked if they had done all their drug protocols. Nobody was saying anything much, just dealing with their own part of the business. The energy on all of them showed me clearly that they had given up. This was over and they knew it. I was dead.

I walked around my bed, through the people in the room. I looked at Bernie as I moved by him. His face was expressionless, with that blank look that people in shock have. I stroked his face as I moved past him.

Focused now, I found my body and looked at it. It looked small, cold and lifeless. There is dullness to a dead body and a flatness to it that no matter how hard you try, as a living person you cannot emulate. It is as if every ounce of willpower and depth has departed and you are now truly just an empty vessel. For a few seconds I wondered if I could make it back into my body. Would there be enough of me left in the cells for me to reinvigorate? I did not know, but I was determined to try. There was a momentary sense of revulsion to that thought, of stepping back into that thing lying there, like the thought of stepping into cold jelly.

Determined, I stepped forward and into my body, connecting first to my feet. It felt like cold glue had swirled around my ankles and I was able to sink down, turning around and falling/floating back into my body. I could feel my body grasping my energy and pulling my energy in.

It was as simple as that. I would probably like to write about trumpets and noise, or special rituals, but there was none of that. It was actually quite peaceful and simple. From there I connected fully to my body, lying back and settling in. I was 'home', feet first. I guess that means that I was a breech birth for my second birth.

The interesting thing was that this time I could enter my body and stay in it. Unlike when I tried to enter my body when I first realized I was dead, this time there was no barrier. It was like glue was bonding me to me, as if even if I did want to leave my body, I could not. I could feel that I was bonded and for the first few moments at least, I was not brain damaged. My body and my brain felt intact and I could feel my chest rise as I struggled for breath. I felt my lungs fill, and, as with my first breath, my lungs burned with the effort and the chemicals that fill oxygen. Then immediately my heart started to beat. Painful, loud in my ears, my heart started to thump against my chest as I came alive.

I could feel the people in the room with me. I could feel their shock; I heard their words as they registered surprise at my sudden and unexpected resurgence.

My body filled with pain. I could feel my crushed chest. I could feel my heart laboring as it struggled to continue to beat. My brain seemed to melt. It felt hot inside my head, almost burning in its intensity. I knew that the physical brain damage was connecting to my consciousness, telling my consciousness which parts it could use and which parts were off limits.

To the paramedics who were watching, my heart and my breathing started at the exact same moment. It was, they told me; just like I had decided to live and back I had come. Just like that.

"She's breathing!" one of the firemen said loudly.

"I have a heartbeat!" another exclaimed almost at the same time. They were excited. For one of the firemen, this was his first 'save' in 12 years. Immediately, the pain was all-encompassing. I could not breathe; it felt as if my chest was being crushed and all I could physically feel was pain and noise. Every part of my body began to buzz and burn. There was not a place that did not hurt.

I shrank into a tiny pin-point of light. From that moment on, to the amazement of the firemen/paramedics from the Metropolitan Fire Brigade, and the ambulance officer from MAS, I was alive.

Carmel Bell

The journey continues

When I next became aware four days had passed. I do not remember the ambulance trip to the hospital, or having drips inserted into my body when I got there. No memories remain of being intubated, except for when I swallow food. I can only imagine that being intubated was very uncomfortable and as I still have some body memory from that event, I am grateful that I do not remember it.

I can also remember almost nothing of the drug induced coma that I was placed into, other than darkness and a sense of entombment, nor do I remember them cooling my body to help save my brain. Every time I swam to the surface I was pulled back down and away from anything coherent. It was a nightmare. I would guess that a natural coma is a much more pleasant event, but again, I am grateful that they placed me into the coma, as it allowed me to heal.

When I struggle, really struggle, I can get a sense of complete darkness from that time, and muffled sounds but I cannot work out what the sounds mean. Logic tells me that it must be the sounds of machines, and cleaners moving around, sounds of doctors talking over me, people visiting me, crying and being in shock. Perhaps it was even the sounds of silence, the sounds of Bernie sitting next to me, hour upon hour, worrying about leaving me in case I woke up, or died and also worried about our children, left at home, alone. I can sometimes remember a delicate whisper of touch across my skin, a gentle stroking of me, mostly on my right hand but I cannot remember responding to that touch, or even feeling like I wanted to respond. I was there, in my body, but I was also a million miles away. I have no knowledge, no clue, not even a theory as to where my consciousness might have been during that time. It was simply not where my body was.

I can sometimes recall coming into my body and then I would be aware of disjointed feelings or events. I can recall feeling a tear on my face but I am unable to respond. I am utterly and completely unable to do anything other than lie there passively.

I know that I was aware of some discomforts. When I swim to the surface I can claw out some memories of things like the tube that was down my throat to intubate me being gently maneuvered. I can feel drips being placed into my arms or wiggled, a catheter being inserted into my groin. I can feel liquids churning through my veins and sometimes I feel coldness, and always I feel a heat throughout my chest and my brain. My brain is burning and it is from that which I retreat.

I remember only one conversation during that time, between Bernie and my best friend, Allan. This was just before I woke up from the coma.

Allan and Bernie were talking about how the intensivist had told Bernie to find a nursing home for me. I was expected to never be independent again. His response to that prognosis had been simply "You don't know Carmel." No more, no less.

I can recall only the feeling of these two men at my bedside and those words from Bernie. I could feel his faith in me. I could feel – it was not hope as he did not hope that I would recover. He *knew* that I would.

Between these two realities of life and unconsciousness, I am inside myself running around screaming. I am scared and overwhelmed. I have no conscious idea of where I am, how I got there or how I was going to get back. In my memories, the closest description I can give is to say it was like the ghost train rides. I am steaming along, in blackness, on a bumpy, uncomfortable ride, with shrieks echoing around me, and faces, horrors, leaping out of places suddenly, bloodless, headless monstrosities, screaming at me. No warning, no respite, no kindness, no laughter, just unrelenting, unforgiving blackness, noise, sorrow.

I am alive.

Using Metatronic Energy

I can feel…something. It is a pain, a heat, a hurt, something. I am not sure *where* in my body that something is. I hear voices, a murmur, and then words but just a few.

"…never walk or talk again…"

"…day four is as good as it usually gets…"

"…nursing home…"

Breathing hurts. It more than hurts, it is as if every ounce of oxygen that I struggle to pull in to my lungs is thick and empty. I can feel dizziness in my head, uncomfortable and destabilizing. I am nauseous but my body feels strangely empty and I know that I am not going to throw up.

I want to scream in agony but…I cannot. I find that strange and I struggle to orientate myself. It is as if I am swimming only to have been dumped by a wave and I am unsure of which way is up. Then I am momentarily distracted by the realization that nothing seems to work. I cannot move, I cannot scream, I cannot roll. My head is spinning but my back is still. I cannot feel my legs, but I am aware of tubes and I feel like I am a Borg from Star Trek, part of the collective.

Then back to pain. My eyes won't open. Nothing works. I know I am in trouble. I *know* I am in Trouble. Capital T. But why I am in trouble I do not know. All I can feel is pain and all I can remember are those few words, "…never walk or talk again…"

It all fades. Then comes crashing back, like a wave hitting me with a crushing *ROAR!* I feel the sound, the awareness, the pain crash into my skull. It is angry, hungry, demanding and blinding. Blinding! Even now I struggle to not vomit as I remember it. I feel my body reacting to the pain that I was feeling, inside and outside me. Dizzy, lost, nauseous and off balance. There is light, sound, pressure. Pain. Oh God! I want to cry, scream. Help. I need help! But there is nothing in the dark. There is no-one. I don't even know who I am. Or where I am. I am caught in a giant wave that is rolling me around, scraping me on the bottom of a seabed; I struggle to breathe, to find the way up. There is no 'up', there is no way out, and there is no sound but too much noise. My heart, beating slowly, is pumping against my chest. It is my own tsunami.

I have never felt such violence of my body, such fear.

I am alive. I am human. I am.

I know that time is passing. I know I have breathed and moved and cried without opening my eyes or even waking up.

I hear voices again. I know the voices and I feel – joy? Something. Overwhelmed, I feel something again and I struggle to open my eyes. Nothing happens. Nothing responds to my commands no matter how much I struggle. But I can still hear because a voice drifts in.

"...she wouldn't ever be happy like this..."

"...trapped..."

And I think, loudly and clearly, screaming into my brain. 'I want to be back.' I don't even know where 'back' is. Memories float in. Disjointed. Blackness. Memories of talking to some man. I remember Bernie. I recognize the other voice - my best friend, Allan. I know they are talking about the possibility of me surviving like this. Like this? I reel emotionally and then I fade again.

I can feel grief. Not from me, but from the people speaking. I want to cry, howl, rant, and kick my legs, punch and claw. I am mad. I am madder than that. I am so angry I can barely breathe with the feeling but I still cannot move. This time I fight the urge to slip away again. It is like a huge black cavern and it calls me. It is peaceful and it is calm in that space, and here where I am now, the light hurts and burns my eyelids. Each breath feels as if there are a hundred knives stabbing into me. It feels like all my insides are being crushed and pulverized inside me. Yet still I breathe. Yet still I fight that cavern. I want to reach out.

I search through my mind and my mind burns. What can I find? Children. I had children. Like counting toes I count them in my mind. One, two, three, four. Four children. With each thought my awareness increases a little more. Each thought seems to be pulling me further into this body. With each thought the pain in my body increases but I still have no idea as to why it hurts, or why I cannot feel it.

I am forcing my brain and my body to respond. I am forcing it and I will not relent. I tell it what I want. There are two of me in here, there is me who is thinking and there is me who is the physical brain, the body, the muscles and the tissue. That part of me wants to give up. *'Coward!'* I scream in my head at myself. *'You coward!'*

I slip back into the blackness. It has pulled me down and I can no longer feel my body but now memories swim at me, like sharks from the darkness. They swim at me, hit me and rush away. I can almost feel their blood lust in this madness that I am now locked. Each thought shark drives another memory into my brain or eats one that I could not scoop up to safety before it arrived.

My memories start assaulting me. I can remember talking to someone who said they were Jesus. I also remember now speaking to two of my nephews but these two boys were both dead. I had promised them I would pass messages on to their parents and siblings for them. How had I done this? Where was I when I had done this? They had been happy that I agreed to their request. I struggled now to retain that memory. I knew that it was *important* that I locked this information into my brain. Into a part that was not damaged (?) before I could fade again. I start moving information around in my brain, seeing my brain as a house that had many rooms. I find a room that is clear and I move these memories into there. I can 'see' different areas of my brain lighting up as I begin to think. Thud! Another thought shark slams into my side. I reel. My head hurts.

Other areas of my brain fade quickly to black and disappear. I realize that I am rewiring my brain. Thud! Thud! Thud! Something is pounding me. I can see/feel shark upon shark swimming wildly towards me, pounding, turning, screaming into the blackness, and then charging back at me.

I reached out my hand and I was awake.

I can 'feel' that I am alone and I still could not move much. I can wiggle, just a bit. And I am cold. Frozen cold. I hate the cold, the kind that gets into your bones. This cold feels like it is lodged in my heart, in my brain, in my groin. It feels deep and healing but uncomfortable. I want to shiver but not even that command could illicit a response from my body. I cannot move and already I am exhausted. I can feel the cold in my brain and after the heat that I had been feeling, this was a welcome cold.

I trace the patterns inside my brain. I can feel the damage inside my skull, tender spots that will not work and ache persistently. I try to draw a map in my mind, something for Energy that I am searching for to follow. In the end, I give up and ask only for this Energy to do as it feels it must.

Then I call for Metatronic Energy. To do this is as natural, more natural, than breathing which is now so painful. I can feel the Metatronic Energy I have called as it touches me. Its response is rapid and it feels cool, light, sparkling. I pull it down into my body, drinking it in like water. I feel it warming and moving through my body and cooling as it moves through my brain. It feels like an itch, like a feather being stroked across various parts of my brain and in response, parts of my body start to gently twitch. I feel as Metatronic Energy moves down effortlessly into my heart and then through all my body. Now I shiver. Now I *feel* alive again but still slow, tired. I can feel my brain repairing and I know that I have suffered massive amounts of damage to my brain. I know this just from all the areas that feel numb in my brain.

I know that I should not be able to speak, or walk or be 'normal' ever again. I am alive, but only just, and there is massive, unbelievable grief in me at being alive. This hurts. But I also feel joy because I know that I will again see Bernie and my children. Something is bothering me and I feel around until I can feel tubes in my arms, in my groin. I pull, then pull some more. Pain but they give way and come out. Content because I can feel the energy that I had called working through me I settle down to wait and everything blanks out. My brain feels like a TV that has just been switched off...

...Then something or someone is bothering me. Something is annoying me. I can *feel* the thoughts, the energy directed at me. I feel the annoyance and I struggle to control myself. I start to block the emotions being directed at me but then I feel warmth from them and I let them in. Suddenly Bernie is there. I can feel him and I look at him, pulling myself back into my body. I want to cry. He looks so tired but I have no energy to spare for him. Nothing left to give but hope and love.

I struggle to speak. "I came back for you." My throat is tight, dry. I can feel him reel emotionally, energetically. That is all I have. I can't say anything more and I want to sleep now. His pain hurts too much. I am struggling not to cry.

Then there is nothing.

Chapter Nineteen:

The side effects of Dying

The only therapy that has been used on me to heal my brain after I died was the Metatronic Energy that I used and the staff in ICU lowering my body temperature to 33c before allowing me to warm up again naturally.

I used Metatronic Energy on myself, for myself, as I have described above. All of this is a true story and every part of it can be verified. Medically it is provable that I was dead for at least 45 minutes, observed and recorded by one or more people.

If I wasn't in Heaven, where was I?

When I stood in my cardiologist's office in July of 2009 (five months post death) I asked him if he could explain my recovery. How did I live and then start to heal? My cardiologist said to me "We have no way to explain this, other than your own energy and a miracle."

Waking up

After four days in a medically induced coma, breathing with the aid of a ventilator, I suddenly became aware of myself. I became aware of what was left of me. At first all I was aware of was pain; I couldn't think clearly, I was simply aware that my body wouldn't obey me and that it hurt to breathe. I could hear people speak, feel their presence and their thoughts. I could sense kindness and not kindness. I could dream. When I dreamt I did not dream as a person with brain damage. I dreamed as I was before my death. It was much more peaceful to be asleep but I was also afraid of sleeping because I did not know where I would be when I woke.

As I woke that day, the pain in my chest overwhelmed me and I faded again. My sternum and a couple of ribs had been broken from the CPR. Every breath was agony. I faded in and out until I could not tell the difference between awake and asleep.

Sometimes I heard sounds, but in my ocean of pain, they were often meaningless.

Gradually, I began to pick out words, and phrases.

"…never walk or talk again…"

"…day four is as good as it usually gets…"

"…Nursing home…"

I drifted away, towards a black cavern. I knew that I recognized the voices, and I felt love and joy for whoever these people were, but I couldn't move; the pain was too strong. The drugs that they had me on were probably stronger.

The voices were back.

"…she wouldn't ever be happy like this…"

"…trapped..."

This time, I knew the voices were those of Bernie and my best friend, Allan. I was aware of their emotional state: I felt their deep sadness, and it became my sadness.

At some pre-conscious level I knew what the people who loved me were discussing: whether it would be kinder to allow me to die, rather than live some not-alive, not-dead experience. *I'm alive, and I want to be back!* I thought, but I had no understanding of where "back" might be.

I remember I had spoken with my nephews, who were dead and had I promised to pass on messages to their families. I had spoken to Jesus and Metatron, and I made an agreement, but what was it? I had to remember.

I'd been dead for at *least* 47 minutes, but who knows really how long it was between dying, realizing I was dead. And I had brain damage. I was aware of this too, so I tried to lock my important memories into those parts of my brain which weren't damaged. As I gathered these disjointed memories together I was like someone who's walking through a house wrecked by a bomb blast, picking up the dusty, fragmented treasures of their former life.

Each time when I think back to this time, I feel in my mind a kind of echoing hollowness. There is no particular joy, no sense of belonging. I feel like the caretaker of a house that has been bomb blasted and I am left behind to walk through these shattered rooms, full of things that were once beautiful and are now just a fragmented ruin. I feel grief.

As I was healing my brain, I shuffled memories and action responses around from place to place, trying to find new locations for old tasks. Into this room went my life with Bernie, the room over there my children's childhoods, then my family, my pets, my friends, my college, into another room. Each event, labeled, located and stored. I felt for places in my brain that were blank.

If I could not feel it when I thought, wiggled my toes, blinked my eyes, I used it for storage. If some part of me did not work, I would find another bit of my brain that was okay and I would let that section take over. This is the best as I can describe what I did. The brain that was used for these tasks ordinarily I was letting rest. I was emptying them out so that they could recover without constant pressure.

This was how I repaired brain damage, even though a neurologist may be horrified by my explanation and my experience.

Each thing or event that I remembered pulled me further back into my body, and each layer of myself that I moved back into me, increased my feelings, so that soon all I felt was a bone-deep cold. I've always hated the cold. My brain does not seem to work so well when I am cold and whilst I was in the coma, they had cooled me with icepacks to lower my body temperature so that my brain cells would be preserved whilst I was struggling to heal. I know that I had been cooled to 33c for 24hours and then I had been allowed to warm up naturally but even though that was only for 24 hours, it took months for me to feel warm again. One of the most traumatic parts of the whole experience that I have been through with dying and recovery was the freezing. Even after I should have been warm, my Guides told me that they were keeping me cool to increase the healing in my brain. It was only afterwards, when I was finally nearly healed that I remembered Metatronic Energy doing the same thing, cooling my brain.

It did not matter to me how hot it was inside my house, or outside, I would be shivering and my body would be cool to the touch.

In the middle of a heatwave, in summer, in February 2009 I was crying for a heater in my room!

I knew I was awake. I was not there and then I was there. Life often is just like that. Dead or not dead. Alive or not alive. Happy or not happy. Not awake. Awake. We are a civilization of absolutes.

The first thing I realized with my consciousness was that I was alone. Then I became even more conscious of the cold. I felt as frozen as if I were encased in a block of ice. The deep cold felt as if it was everywhere, in my heart, my brain, and every part of my body. No matter how uncomfortable I was however, I was also aware that the cold was healing me. I wanted to shiver, but my body didn't know how.

Instinctively, I reached out for Metatronic Energy and as this energy came at my command, it felt cool, light, and sparkling. I drew Metatronic Energy deeply into my body, and was as if every thirsty cell drank it in like wonderful, reviving water. The first thing that I did was call the energy that I use, and it came.

The energy moved through my brain and moved throughout my bloodstream and organs. I could feel my brain kicking in, my internal organs repairing and the bones that had been broken in my chest from the extended CPR mending.

I started to shiver. I was feeling alive again, but very weak and tired. I knew that I had suffered massive brain damage – I could feel it. I could feel how it slowed me down and altered the way I thought and how my body behaved. I knew that by rights, I would never be able to walk, talk, or be normal again, in any way. However, I knew that this did not suit me. 'Heal me,' I asked this energy.

Brain damage is exhausting. You only step consciously into your body occasionally. The rest of the time you are off in a dream world. People swim in and swim out. You are minding your own business, dreaming away, when suddenly it will feel like an explosion has happened right inside your mind and your face. Someone will be there. Like a monstrosity, they swim into focus. It can be frightening. Then they will disappear. Your life is disjointed and tiring. Thoughts and memories feel like sharks swimming out of the deep to slam into you.

At times I would be talking and forget what I was saying, or who I was talking to. I would forget to chew until I realized that I had food in my mouth. My memory lasted for about five minutes.

With brain damage you are there and then you are 'not there'. You disappear as rapidly as dreams do upon awakening. You may 'sound' sensible and I know I frequently did when I was speaking to people but I was only sensible in that instant. It is like having a montage in your brain and you have to try to make sense out of small snippets of information that you are given at that time. But every situation comes loaded with history, so you never really get it. It is a nightmare world.

Over the following days Metatronic Energy continued to move through my body and I continued to heal. At the time that I died, I had been exclusively using, teaching, and passing Metatronic Energy on to others for at least 25 years. Reaching out for it as I started to wake up was, fortunately, completely natural to me.

Think of Metatronic Energy as being like sunlight. After being dead for 47 minutes, my body and brain were severely damaged. The doctors told Bernie that I had suffered massive brain damage. They told him to find a nursing home as they doubted that I would have any kind of normal life. They still look at me as if I'm some kind of miracle, or worse, something that they could not explain and yet, could also not deny.

I got used to medical people who saw me while I was in my coma later looking confused when I spoke to them as I continued to recover. One doctor, the intensivist and I did not even know that there was such a profession did not recognize me. This was the man who had told Bernie to find a nursing home for me. I thank him for his honesty and his compassion and I will repeat again the words Bernie said to him. "You don't know Carmel."

I can't speak too much about the time after I first woke up and spoke to Bernie because thankfully, most of that has been taken from me. I have only flashes of my time in my mind. I have vague memories of my brother, Mark, sitting next to me and reading Spike Milligan to me. Sometimes one of my sisters will float in and then disappear again. Brain damage prevailing, my life became a series of surprises. I would be sitting quietly when something would drag me away from my inner world and I would usually hear the end of a sentence, or a question. This would usually not make any sense to me at all and I would answer as best I could before disappearing back into whatever make-believe world I had been in.

I remember one day of being aware that I was in a bed in a room with four hospital beds in it. I was in the bed on the right hand side of the room, closest to the nurse's station and the other three beds had old men in them. I was lying huddled in a ball on my stomach, watching a small DVD player. The movie I was watching was Audrey Hepburn and Humphrey Bogart in *Sabrina*. I wonder how many times I watched that movie? End of flash.

As time progressed I became aware that there were two of me, the sensible Carmel that I have always known and then this slightly strange and completely bizarre other being that walked huddled over, spun in circles and went "Uh oh," every time she was startled. This creature that I had become could not put two colours together if her life depended on it, or speak sensibly, or drive, or walk. I felt trapped inside my body with this being. I was horrified by this new me. It was a nightmare, a living, breathing hell to be like this. I had little or no self control, no understanding of what to do or how to behave. I was short tempered, impulsive and very touchy. In short, I was brain damaged.

As I healed I learned from other NDE survivors, in particular Nanci Danison, the author of 'Backwards' that there are two consciousnesses inside us because we are a separate race from our bodies. That made sense to me and explained why I kept functioning even when I stepped away from me. It explained why I would act in ways that were childish and immature and yet I still seemed like myself.

Even if I did not want to react or misbehave to a situation, my reaction would happen before I had a chance to stop it. It felt as if there was another being inside my body and that I was the passenger instead of the driver. I would do things, say things and behave in ways that were completely alien to me and yet still seem like me, because I was me, but another me. The animal part, as I have explained, was in control whilst Carmel was away healing.

During this time I behaved in ways that I have never behaved before, or since. All I could do was ask people who had witnessed my behaviour to do me the great kindness of never mentioning it again. Even now it pains me to think of myself at that time.

Emotionally, I was engulfed by grief at being alive; however, I was also conscious of joy, at being able to be with the people I love once more. It was just so hard! I have never felt such intense, enormous, engulfing and personal pain as I felt when I first woke up. If I was not in a non-place, not really thinking, I was in grief. I could not stand people to be near me as I had no psychic protection. I felt as they felt, and as a result I was torn asunder. Even when I had been lying on a bed in ICU, semi comatose I could feel the pain or discontent of the staff and patients around me, but I could not talk to ask for help. I was a prisoner in my own body. I was angry at myself for coming back. I was angry at Bernie for being the reason I came back. I was angry with my children for also being reasons and I found that I needed to keep away from them, so that they would not feel my emotions.

I would swing between crying and being absent. With a memory span of less than five minutes long. I can't imagine the patience that Bernie must have exhibited for me.

My children tell me that whenever I came home on the weekends, during that period of time, I wanted to watch an Owen Wilson film called *"Drill Bit Taylor."* Apparently they are all sick of it but I still can't remember the film.

Six weeks of my life, at least, was consumed by brain damage and I am lucky that this is all I lost. Most people who suffer severe brain damage only manage to claw back a little of themselves.

The time that has completely vanished into the darkness, I am happy to let go. I do not think that I want to remember most if not all of that time. I have the medical records that I have procured to tell me how I was.

My guides tell me that although they locked off sections of my brain and built new pathways for me, all this takes time when you are trying to be human. They had to 'move' many things around to let me function. They also had to allow part of my consciousness to rest and to do so they allowed my 'body consciousness' to be in charge for a while.

But then I found myself at home once again, wondering what I was doing there. I felt completely out of place. I felt that I did not belong anywhere. I was lost and it was up to me alone to sort through all of this and find out who I was and what I wanted to be. As I was, I certainly was not good for anything. I know that people consider it a kindness to work to keep brain damaged people alive, but sometimes that is a cruelty beyond bearing. Every moment can be startling, and every noise can sound like a minefield in your head. There is very little to smile about.

Who are you when you are no longer who you thought you are?

I no longer knew who I was. Who are you when you are no longer anybody? People thought that I was Carmel Bell, others thought that I was Carmel, plain and simple, mother, daughter, wife, lover, healer. None of these were correct.

But who was I? Who had I been?

Every thought and almost every moment felt dangerous and unstable. I felt like I was being tricked and trapped. It felt like everyone wanted something from me, something that I did not want to give. I learned to feel afraid of people and for the first time ever, to look for double meanings in peoples words.

All I can think when I recall that time is the nightmare feeling of the place where I was. My consolation was the knowledge that it had to get better.

Life is a minestrone

Bernie picked me up from the Box Hill hospital and drove me home about three weeks after I died. I had signed myself out of the hospital, but I don't know why I did that, other than I did not feel 'safe' there. I wanted something familiar around me, but I did not recognize anywhere, or anything.

"Where were you?" I had said to Bernie when he arrived to collect me; "I've been waiting..." We were silent for most of the trip home, with me trying to stay stable and upright, with all the movement around me.

I walked through the front door of what I had been told was my home, bracing myself for the likely onslaught. My three youngest children were bound to be pleased to see me. I hoped. I had not seen them for weeks. Not that I could recall.

I stepped through the front door, into the lounge-room. The door shut behind me with a soft thump. I looked back at it and stood still. The word 'breathe' is written on my door. I waited and I breathed.

I was home. I was a stranger in a strange land.

I looked around me again. There was no one there to greet me and I am not sure how I felt. Relieved or disappointed? Neither? I think I felt gratefully indifferent. Bernie had come in behind me and now he dropped my bags on the floor inside the door. Together we stood there, shoulder to shoulder, but not touching. It seemed like a lifetime since I had been here last and I did not recognize most of the house. I felt a slight sense of sorrow and resentment well up in me at the realisation that Bernie had altered the house so much in my absence, but I quickly pushed that feeling down.

"I love what you've done. It looks nice," I said softly. I could feel Bernie next to me, standing silently.

"What do you mean?" he finally asked.

I walked forward into the house without answering. It was only as my memory repaired that I realized that the house was exactly the same. I just could not remember it and Bernie would have been quite confused by my reaction.

My brain was still not working properly. How could it? In such a short space of time and yet here I was expecting me to be normal and feeling angst that I was not. I could walk and talk, often just barely because of the vestibular damage so it felt like I was walking on a rolling ship, all the time. I felt quite unstable and often nauseous from the constant rocking and rolling of the ground that I was on. The motion in my brain and having to brace myself against that motion all the time exhausted me. Even when I was lying down the world was moving. Constant motion is exhausting.

I also no longer knew very much about myself. I felt like a stranger in a strange land. I did not know what colours I liked, or what food I wanted. Actually, everything tasted like cardboard. I have heard people say that before and I never understood that food could actually taste like cardboard. And because I had trouble swallowing, most of what I was given to eat choked me. I was learning to exist on French fries. They were easy to chew, easy to swallow and also had lots of oils in them that I seemed to be craving. Bernie was so busy that he would often forget to help me find food and as I had no urge to find food myself, I could go for a fair length of time without eating before my body would demand sustenance.

I have collected vintage clothes for years and I loved them, the colours, the textures, the beautiful patterns and fabrics. Now I had no interest in them at all. I could not read as I could not concentrate on anything and I no longer knew what I wanted to read anyway.

For some unknown reason, I had discharged myself from hospital, and I was awaiting entry into the rehabilitation hospital, so I felt like a guest in my home. I felt like I did not belong here. I could still feel Metatronic Energy working in my brain but it was pretty obvious to everybody, including myself, that I was just a long way off normal.

I stayed home for that weekend before going to the Royal Talbot Hospital. I can remember during that weekend picking our daughter up from my parents. We met them at a shopping centre but all I can remember is how hard it was to be there, in that place, with all the people around me, all the noise and electronics bombarding me, things rushing at me, and having to sit and wait for my parents and my daughter to appear. I wanted to spin in circles, I wanted to walk around and buy things, but who knew what, or what for?

But everything I purchased in that time, which was more than I needed to, was a mistake. I had no idea what I was doing and what I was buying. Fortunately, I did not carry a bag or a wallet. I did not even remember that I needed those things, so what I could buy was very limited.

Into the Talbot

I don't remember much of the rehab hospital either. I can really only remember the last week of rehab. I remember waking up one morning and opening my eyes. Immediately I could see a small notice on the side of my bed side table. It said "On the 15th of February 2009 you had a cardiac arrest and you were dead for 47 minutes..." I was shocked. I had no idea! And apparently I had no idea the day before, and the day before that, and I would also have no idea tomorrow! It's funny now, but at the time it broke Bernie's heart.

One time Bernie could not make it in to see me until late in the day and when he came in he found me talking to the blowflies. 'It's okay,' I told him, 'The flies were keeping me company.'

After my death I found that I had the ability to hear animals and to understand them, from flies, to birds, to cats and dogs. The birds would not fly away from me when I walked up to them. That gift has gradually eased. It was actually quite nice to just sit and listen to the conversation flying through the air. Not that they had much to say, but still, it was soothing.

And now I was being discharged from the rehab hospital.

I was upset when Bernie finally arrived to pick me up because the doctors who were supervising me whilst I was in there had come to see me before I went home and they had gone through all their protocols, warning me not to be alone, to be careful when I was cooking, that I was not allowed to drive and that many marriages fail such an event as brain damage. They gave me statistics about the percentage of failures. From their delivery of this news, I am certain that all or many of these doctors could be Aspergers.

But what did I hear? That the marriage that I had rejected heaven for was likely to fail. I was handed an envelope that contained details for a marriage and family counselling service and then they left.

I waited until they were gone and then I cried. I wanted my marriage to last.

I suppose that they needed to tell me these things, but I did not need to hear them just then. But what else could they do but warn me? No system is perfect and rehabilitation is no different. I am grateful to these doctors for being there.

Healing Vestibular imbalance

Home at last, six weeks after my cardiac arrest, brain damaged, in love with Bernie and a mother to four children. I also had a college that I had not been near for months, despite trying to get there. I believe that one of the first questions I had asked Bernie was about the college and the students, worrying about them and their progress. He assured me that some of my graduates from previous years had stepped up to take over for Bernie and me so that the college could keep running. I was amazed and grateful at how much care that they had taken with my new students, and how much of the knowledge that I had taught my graduates they had remembered and been able to pass on.

Thanks to these people, I was able to return home and leave the college for them to run, still, giving me time to rebuild. If I could have found a corner I would have crawled into it. Bernie and the children kept pulling me out of the corner.

I had no idea who I was still. None at all.

I was already a Medical Intuitive, but I no longer knew if that was what I should be doing, or if this was what I wanted to be doing. I was lost, utterly lost. I was in so much emotional pain that I was stunned.

I remember Jesus and Metatron asking me to teach Metatronic Energy to people, but I wish that they had sent me a postcard and not given me a ticket home.

And I was scared. I did not fit in, no matter what I did. I was scared that I had made a mistake in coming back, that Heaven would be angry with me for rejecting it and would never allow me back. I was scared that my presence would harm my children or Bernie. It took me a few days of wallowing before I decided that enough was enough. If Heaven wanted me, Heaven could come and collect me!

The vestibular imbalance that I had woken up with was still a problem and it was wearing me out. I was distressed on a daily basis, not to mention exhausted by the constant rocking motion of my world. I would go to see Janet, the physiotherapist at the Royal Talbot and she would give me exercises to do, to try and ease the condition. They helped but they did not get rid of it. If you are always rocking, it makes it very hard to get up from a chair, out of a bed, out of a car, or off the back of a motorbike. Vestibular imbalance affects everything.

Janet taught Bernie to place his hand on the top of my head if I was really dizzy, to give me some spatial awareness again, but this was only a temporary measure. I knew that I would not be able to go back to work like this.

Then one day I was completely exhausted and close to defeat. I stomped down my hallway to my bedroom, determined to lie down and ignore the world. I flung myself on to the bed and announced to the world and anyone else who cared to listen, "I've had enough! This has got to stop!" I firmly closed my eyes and held them shut. It was about 2.30pm and the room was darkened, but not blacked out. I was feeling quite alone when a voice said next to me, quietly, 'Open your eyes.' Surprised, I did, and standing next to me, next to my bed, was Hiram, one my guides. Hiram is my primary healer. He smiled at me and reached out his hand, placing it on the top of my head, just like Bernie would do when he was trying to stop the spinning in my brain.

I was lying in my bed, with Hiram's hand on the top of my head, speechless. I could feel the weight of his hand, the pressure of his hand on me, but there was no physical warmth. I looked into his eyes, and he looked into mine. I could see concern, compassion and love in his eyes. I remembered our time together, and I knew how much energy it must be taking Hiram to be here, doing this. Then I blinked and Hiram was gone.

So was the vestibular imbalance.

I got up, standing to my feet. The world stayed still. I started to cry, for many reasons, not the least of which was gratitude for this incredible soul who has traversed so many times and so many places with me, who has loved me in our shared past and who loves me now.

I have been lucky to have such love in my lives, not once, but twice.

Rebuilding my life

It was now nearly eight months since my death. If I was a baby, I would be almost ready to be birthed.

I felt lost as to what my date of birth should be – the original date or the day I died? Or both dates? And would that have me aging twice as fast? In one of our 'side' conversations, Jesus told me that I would be sent back younger than I was. Is there a market for this in the beauty industry, I wondered? I could walk, cook and clean. I was struggling with organisation but I was back to work at my college, teaching, even though that was exhausting.

I was also in my clinic again, seeing clients. I could still 'do' this, with remarkable speed and accuracy, even better than before. Seeing energy was an easy job, hearing my guides as natural as hearing a human, but my shields against other people were still not strong. But I knew that it was only a matter of time for me to get back to normal.

But the question kept coming back to me, 'Is this what I wanted to do?' Not because I did not believe in it, because I did, I do, even more than before. I can see clearly and show you clearly just how effective this energy is. I am alive and working again because of it.

And because of Metatronic Energy, every day my brain improves in huge leaps and bounds. Every day I become more and more normal. If only I had back the boundless energy that I had before, the inspiration and determination that I had before, I would be happy.

I have struggled with the need to be 'healthy'. I have this argument in my mind that tells me to eat sensibly, not to drink, and to exercise, and then I say to myself 'Yeah? Why? Did that and I died!'

Even so, I eat, drink and exercise.

My body is almost normal again. Nearly all of the brain damage is also gone. But who am I?

Then nine months post death and we have just celebrated my birthday. I was surprised by how indifferent I felt to my birthday. I was not really expected to reach this mark. My heart has been battered and bruised from all the compressions it underwent, and also from stopping in the first place. Then from surgery to implant a pacemaker in case it happens again. My poor, overworked heart. The pacemaker hurts. It is painful to roll onto my side and painful to do pushups or pec decs. Still, I am happy to have one.

Will I ever have this happen to me again? My Guides say 'No', but I sometime worry about waking up dead once more, but what would I do about it if I did? Would I come back or would I choose to stay dead this time?

The medical outlook is that I am lucky if I survive 12 months post death. Yeah. 'You don't know Carmel,' Bernie would say to that. He would set his face and he would say that.

There are so many questions and most of them are unanswerable questions.

I am rebuilding more every day. Hiram helped to repair the vestibular imbalance and who knows what else. I can't really say conclusively what was wrong with my brain due to brain damage, because I had a global brain injury. Global brain injury puts damage right throughout your brain and not just in one section. The damage that shows up can be unpredictable and severe in some parts, nonexistent in others.

No-one could tell me what was wrong or what was likely to be wrong, or likely to get back to being right. The doctors did not know what killed me, they did not know what saved me and they did not know what repaired my brain or my body. Some of the things that they wrote about me in my files were cruel and intolerant and the kind of things that you would hope that people in the medical world would never think or say, but they did.

I think that 'they' expected me to be 'normal'. For a 47-year-old Asperger, with brain damage, I was normal. Most people who are 'normal' are only 'normal' because they are pretending, acting, appearing to be socially acceptable. Everybody has shocking thoughts, risqué thoughts and destructive thoughts. The vast majority of people hide these thoughts from everybody, even their closest friends.

Part of my job, my skills, is to read the hidden parts of people's brains.

I sometimes think back to the time when I was in Box Hill Hospital and I am grateful to the staff and the patients who were there with me. I don't know the names of the elderly gentlemen who were in the room with me in Box Hill Hospital but I wish I did so that I could thank them. They looked after me with exceptional kindness and protectiveness. They cared for me as if I was one of their own. I was safe with them. Thank you, gentlemen.

I reviewed my brain after Hiram healed the vestibular imbalance. What was wrong with it? Sometimes it was balance, sometimes motivation then decision making, then inspiration, then speech, words, thoughts, numbers and more. My problems seemed to change rapidly.

Sometimes it is just energy levels. I am too tired to do anything and then suddenly I am full of life and struggling to slow down.

The part that I find amusing, for want of a better description, is my sudden strange desire to smoke. I used to smoke, years ago, but not very much. Hardly anyone realized that I smoked, but since I woke up from the coma I have had this strange, compelling desire to smoke. In hospital I used to follow the smokers around.

I gave up smoking without intending to. One night I was just sitting outside, quietly having a smoke when out of my mouth came the words, "I will never smoke again." I was surprised and I immediately thought, 'yeah, sure.' But I put out the cigarette and went inside the house.

I have never smoked since. Not once, not even the sneak, when you are drunk, smoke. Never. I did not use the nicotine gum either. I just went cold turkey, which was the hardest thing I have ever done.

It does not bother me being around smokers, smelling them, holding them, or anything like that. I am not the reformed bore about it. I just don't do it.

So here I was, months after dying, home again. Reasonably stable on my feet, lost, grief struck and wondering who I was and why I had come back to Earth.

Healing the brain

Ten months post death. I still had several issues with my brain that needed repair. I wanted to be as normal as possible as fast as possible. I also knew that there was no medical field where you could go and get help with repairing the brain. The help that is offered is actually pretty useless. It pretty much consists of sitting back and waiting, letting time do the job.

However, I have never been up for the 'let's wait and see' philosophy. The way I deal with these issues is to identify the problem and then use Metatronic Energy on my brain to rewire the pathways. That is what I am doing. I'm rewiring my brain and the neural pathways. I wish that I could do this for everyone who is brain injured.

One of the toughest challenges that I have had to face in my career as a healer is the simplicity of what I do. It is ridiculously simple to use this energy and to heal with it. As you can see, even a person with brain damage can do it, so how hard can it be?

The difficulty actually lies in the fact that humans like to complicate things and mess things up. Humans do not like simple. Humans like secret symbols and rituals and routines that they have to be 'initiated' into. It makes them feel 'special'.

Again and again, when I teach people, I have to keep pulling them back and reining them in and telling them to stop complicating it.

Keep it simple. Keep it the way Metatron wanted it. Simple.

Trust me, he would not have chosen me if he wanted complicated. I walk away from anything and anybody that becomes complicated. I just don't have the attention span to deal with it otherwise. And I get bored. Easily. In fact the best asset in your healing kit is the ability to get bored.

I ask all my clients to get bored with the game they are playing and when they achieve that, I know we are on the home stretch.

Are you bored with your ill health yet?

Prognosis for the rest of my life

I am still healing. Every day I feel more shifts in my brain, more repairs, more leaps forward. I direct these leaps with my intent and Energy.

In December 2009 I sat in the Royal Talbot talking to the rehabilitation doctor about my injury and my progress when this doctor said to me "You know, we have done nothing for you. You have done it all yourself." And he was right. There is no way to heal a brain for someone else. And the only energy I have ever seen – ever- that has healed a brain is Metatronic Energy.

Chapter Twenty:

The Journey home

Questions, facts and some answers.

Some questions and answers about dying and death. These are the most common questions that I have been asked.

Did you know you were going to die?

Yes, but I did not believe it.

Does everyone know that they are going to die?

I *believe* that they do. In most NDErs there is a strong theme that comes through when you ask them questions about how messages about dying started to come to them in the time before they died. For me, it was the constant hearing of a song by a band called Faker – 'This Heart Attack'.

Also it is quite common to find that many of these people start to clean up their belongings – getting rid of things – reconnecting or apologising to people.

Did it hurt to die?

The short answer for me is no, but I can't answer for everybody because I think that, logically, being run over or stabbed would hurt. Fortunately the body would go into shock and the shock would fix that. So, no, the actual dying would not hurt. It did not hurt me.

In terms of the soul leaving the body, no, that did not hurt. There was absolutely no pain, no discomfort to be felt when leaving the body.

Why didn't you see the Light?

I asked that myself. I felt kind of duped at the time and so I asked the question. I was told that people who are *not meant to* stay dead will see the light and the tunnel and that this was the 'waiting room' for heaven. It is kind of like a barrier that you can look over but not go through. These people who see the light would not enter into actual heaven proper. This was not because they weren't allowed to, or were not good enough; it was because heaven is harder to return from.

Did it hurt to re-enter the body?

No, it did not hurt. Once I got close enough to my body I really had no choice. Upon reflection I felt a bit like a fly caught in a Venus fly trap. It was like it trapped me and in there I stayed. I believe that this is how souls stay inside the body in the first place, even when they are astral travelling.

Did you enter in through the Crown Chakra?

No – I did not. I entered through my feet, or more fully, that was the first place that I connected to, then I just lay back into my body.

How did it feel when you re-entered? Was it like you were being born?

It didn't feel like I was being born. At first I felt like I was sinking into my body, perhaps like it was quicksand and then I felt heavy all of a sudden. Once I was back inside and I was in my brain again, I could feel all the damage that had happened to me. Before that moment, there was no damage that I could feel. I was completely disattached from my body until I decided to re-enter it.

Coming back to life was interesting. I had tried to lie down into my body before I went to heaven and I was literally repulsed by my body. But once I was allowed to leave heaven and go back to my room, it was like my body had been waiting for me. The paramedics had certainly kept it warm, with the blood circulating so that it was in reasonable condition to re-enter.

I am very grateful that they were there; doing that for me, because I dispute that anyone could heal a body or a brain that had been properly dead for quite some time.

How did I heal myself?

I used Metatronic Energy to heal myself. That is all I used. Afterwards, I followed my own guideline of searching for the reasons, grounding, sealing, and then dumping. There were no side lines of drugs that I don't want to mention, or other healers coming along to give me a hand. All other healers were blocked, from right around the world. I do not like unrequested healing. I won't send it and I won't accept it.

I did have surgery to implant a pacemaker and the pacemaker still sits, unused, in my chest. I am happy to have it, but I am quite certain that I do not need it.

I wish that I could tell you that I did this, or did that, but I did nothing apart from call energy in. I have done this, using Metatronic Energy, with other people and it has worked for them also. Once I have it clear in my head what it is I want to do, I call Energy in and it is done. This is what I call Medical Intuition. The energy itself is easy to use, but it gets its strength from knowing the pathways that we are trying to repair or clear.

Learning Metatronic Energy

The best way to learn is in person from someone like me. Can you find it on your own? Maybe. Maybe not. Some people have, like me, but most find an energy frequency that is denser, more like Reiki. My family was wired to use Metatronic Energy, so there has always been someone in my family, in every generation, who has worked as a healer and has passed Metatronic Energy on. This time round it was my turn.

What does a Medical Intuitive do?

A Medical Intuitive will scan your energy field – your aura and your chakras – for the true cause of any symptoms you are experiencing, whether these symptoms are physical, emotional or spiritual. They will use their intuition and their guidance to do this. The easiest analogy is to imagine that a Medical intuitive is like and MRI or a CT that can read the physical body, the energetic body and the emotional body.

Any illness will show up as a block or an energy 'glitch' in your field. An experienced Medical Intuitive will have read a sufficient number of people's fields that they are able to discern what they are seeing and what it means.

To me, illnesses show up as different coloured clouds around people. These clouds are as diffuse as water that has food dye in it and then washed lightly over glass. They are soft and hard to see unless you are aware what it is you are looking for.

All illnesses have their root cause in an emotional area. This is why most people consult a Medical Intuitive and this is why a Medical Intuitive will talk to you about the emotional issues in your life. They are looking for the pathways into you that have caused the blocks.

In addition, a complete scan by a Medical Intuitive will also reveal any weaknesses in your body and your spirit that will allow illnesses to be experienced by you. The ultimate aim of the Medical Intuitive is to prevent illness in you and to help balance any that is currently there.

Why would you use a Medical Intuitive?

You may already have an illness that you want to discover more about such as the emotional reason behind your illness, or where and how it may be progressing. Or you may be feeling as if something is not quite right, or you may just be wishing for a check-up. A Medical Intuitive is a preventative service as well as a foreseeing service

A Medical Intuitive, such as me is also a healer. I will diagnose the condition and then I will take steps to decrease the condition or to make the condition defunct.

I will do this through the use of Metatronic Energy, which is a much higher level energy than previously used. It removes the stories from the body that have caused the condition or problem.

Do I have to believe in it for it to work?

No. No more than you need to believe that an x-ray machine will work. You are energy and energy can be read.

Even if your beliefs are different to my beliefs, you can still be successfully read and gain tremendous insight and benefit from a session.

Do you train people to be a Medical Intuitive?

Yes, I do. But I do not train them through a book. This book was written to help people understand Medical Intuition and to equip them to know whether they might want to try it as a client, or learn to do it as a practitioner.

Are all Medical Intuitives the same?

No. They are all different. This book is about how I work and how the people I have trained work. A large percentage of the Medical Intuitives in Australia have been trained by me through my Funshops, or my college, but not all of them have been. The ones that have not been work in their own way, so I cannot tell you how they work, or what their background and training is. I expect people that I train to be taught anatomy and physiology, to have compassion, integrity, insight and a good connection with their guides. I am also a healer. Not all Medical Intuitives are.

Finale

Remember...

The physical act of healing does not have to be complicated.

The physical act of healing does not take a long time. Just because a healer stands over you for an hour it does not mean that they are more effective than someone who takes five minutes.

Healing will happen when you are ready.

Energy moves in an instant.

It is possible to change how you think and feel.

If you change how you think and feel, you can change the world.

You are the product of every moment of your life, including the cells that went into your creation.

Whether you come to Medical Intuition through interest, through choice as a hopeful practitioner or even as a potential client hoping to discover if this could help you, Medical Intuition is a serious profession, with responsibilities. I have met a lot of people think that the alternative healing professions are easy to go into and easy to do, particularly if you are going to learn an energetic profession such as this.

Some people feel that if it is energy and you can't see it, then you can do anything with it. You can't. Energy itself can be easy to use but it is very hard to master, particularly if you intend to use it to help other people.

Precisely because *it is* energy, how you are in yourself, your thoughts, your feelings, and your involvement in the whole process at the time, will have a large impact on the results. Because of that, these energetic professionals have responsibilities attached. You will often be dealing with vulnerable, scared and sad people and you will *always* be dealing with people who are hoping that you are a solution.

I received an email late last year from a young man who was in therapy for a mental health condition. He wanted to learn Medical Intuition so that he could work, earning money doing healings, whilst being healed. This was not an unusual email and although I do understand his desire, I do not recommend it. His mental condition could alter his perception and not necessarily in a good or helpful way. Because he would be dealing with energy his words and his actions could carry more weight and therefore more disastrous consequences. His journey through the woods may well give him tremendous insight in the future, but not until he is out of the woods.

If you become a Medical Intuitive, people will rely on you and your findings. They will act and react to what you say. They will go to their doctor and say 'A Medical Intuitive told me..."

Intuitive does not mean 'all knowing'. To become a Medical Intuitive is a skill that you should be guided in, with support and training. Being taught does not make you less talented than a person who was born with the skill. Training really only makes you *more* trained. So be taught.

If you are seriously interested, I strongly advise you to take a course in anatomy and physiology, should you wish to pursue Medical Intuition. Also, I recommend that you learn first aid. And a good, well trained Medical Intuitive will have a link to the medical world. They will work closely with medical practitioners. You can only recognize what you understand.

Even if you want to use your intuition for yourself only, become curious and knowledgeable about the body and about the diseases and conditions, particularly about common ailments like Diabetes and heart disease that affect it. If you hear about it, or read about it, take a few minutes to research it. Your attention is being drawn to it for some reason.

A final note:

This is quietly between you and I, for those of you who made it this far. Just a few little inside thoughts. Keep them to yourself because you would not want to be thought of as radical.

Healing is *easy* if you understand what *caused* the illness and you stop trying to be 'fantastic'. Most healers have worked out incredibly complicated systems because they need these systems for *them* to feel good. But all these symbols and hand waving's and mutterings and standing over someone for hours on end are just as real and just as necessary as wearing a fish on your head.

Buy a snapper – it is bigger, has a larger abdominal cavity and will fit on your head nicely.

Your body *wants* to be healthy and balanced.

Energy moves instantly which is *why* you can watch TV or listen to a radio. It does not require sacred symbols, begging, or anything else. It just requires the use thereof.

Healing of the body is not instant because the body cannot tolerate instant healing.

The brain is healable.

Thank you for reading my book, travel well.

Blessings,
Carmel Bell

Index of Exercises

Exercise One:	Seeing energy around trees and plants	101
Exercise two:	Seeing human energy	108
Exercise three	Feeling energy	114
Exercise four:	Grounding	118
Exercise five:	Sealing	120
Exercise six:	Feeling Metatronic energy	130
Exercise seven:	Throwing into the bin	200

Bibliography:

Christopher Brookmyre – A snowball in hell

Derek Landry – Skullduggery Pleasant books

Backwards – Nanci Danison

Coming back to life – PMH Atwater

The big book of near death experiences – PMH Atwater

Caroline Myss – Anatomy of the Spirit

Louise Hays – You can heal your life

Viktor Frankl – Man's search for meaning

Annette Noontil- The body is the barometer of the Soul